THE <u>NEW</u> SELF HELP SERIES
TINNITUS AND CATARRHAL DEAFNESS

A natural, self-help programme to alleviate these distressing complaints and to re-establish a health-promoting life-style.

D1635235

THE <u>NEW</u> SELF HELP SERIES

TINNITUS AND CATARRHAL DEAFNESS

ARTHUR WHITE
N.D., D.O.

THORSONS PUBLISHING GROUP

First published March 1986

© THORSONS PUBLISHING GROUP LIMITED 1986

British Library Cataloguing in Publication Data

White, Arthur
Tinnitus and catarrhal deafness: a natural, drug-
free programme to bring relief and restore health.
1. Tinnitus—Treatment   2. Self-care, Health
I. Title

617.8   RF293.8

ISBN 0-7225-1305-4

*Published by Thorsons Publishers Limited,
Wellingborough, Northamptonshire, NN8 2RQ, England.*

Printed in Great Britain by
Richard Clay Limited, Bungay, Suffolk.

5   7   9   11   13   12   10   8   6

Contents

Note to reader

Before following the self-help advice given in this book readers are earnestly urged to give careful consideration to the nature of their particular health problem, and to consult a competent physician if in any doubt. This book should not be regarded as a substitute for professional medical treatment, and whilst every care is taken to ensure the accuracy of the content, the author and the publishers cannot accept legal responsibility for any problem arising out of the experimentation with the methods described.

1.

Start at the Beginning

Whenever we are faced with a difficult problem it is always a sound policy to start at the beginning and work systematically through the various aspects until we reach a logical and satisfactory solution. The problem with which this book is concerned is a very distressing one — i.e. *tinnitus*, which in turn is almost invariably associated with some degree of *catarrhal deafness*.

In their anxiety to find a solution to their problems many readers of a book of this kind are tempted to glance down the list of contents and, ignoring the preliminary chapters, turn immediately to the section wherein a plan of treatment is disclosed. The temptation to do this is perfectly natural and understandable but it should be resisted, because if any treatment regime is to be effective it is essential that the reader should understand not only what he is required to do but *why* he is doing it. Therefore, having persuaded the reader to restrain his or her natural desire to embark as soon as possible on the road that may lead to salvation from the misery of head-noises and deafness, let us examine the chain of events which has given

Fise to the existing problem.

Recurring Problems

Although the sufferer is probably middle-aged or elderly, there is little doubt that for many years — and possibly even from childhood — there has been a history of recurring colds and influenza, as well as coughs, tonsillitis and the myriad other catarrhal afflictions which, unfortunately, are widely regarded as inevitable concomitants of present-day life.

The fact is that these recurring upsets are only inevitable because they are made so by the mode of living imposed by our parents during our formative years and accepted without question — or even thought — as we pass through the various stages of development and reach adult status.

For many of us, the process started with bottle-feeding in infancy when, either because of domestic expediency or as a result of misguided advice from a doctor or welfare clinic, breast-feeding was abandoned early, or perhaps not even attempted, and replaced by a mixture of cow's milk and refined and sweetened cereals. Today, fortunately, there is wide recognition of the fact that breast-fed babies have an appreciably higher degree of natural immunity from infectious illness than those who are fed on cow's milk and proprietary infant foods. Indeed, cow's milk has been indicted as a major causative factor in asthma and infantile eczema, and it is common practice to exclude dairy products from the diet of victims of these very distressing disorders.

The harm caused by this early nutritional error is further compounded by the addition of cane sugar in an attempt to 'humanize' cow's milk, with the result that the infant becomes accustomed to unnaturally sweet foods at a very early age. This predilection for sugary and starchy foods has far-reaching effects as the infant progresses through childhood and adolescence, during which period he is often allowed, and even encouraged, to indulge a perverted taste for sweets, cakes, biscuits, chocolate, white bread, sweetened breakfast cereals and highly coloured beverages which are little more than a dangerous mixture of sugar and water laced with chemical colourings and flavourings.

It is not surprising, therefore, that — since 'the child is father to the man' — by the time maturity is achieved the appetite for these denatured products will have developed to the point of addiction and that life will be punctuated by a succession of colds, coughs, sore throats, tonsillitis, decaying teeth, acne and various other respiratory and skin disorders. Indeed, it is a tribute to the body's extraordinary powers of adaptation and self-preservation that so many of us survive to lead a normal active life — at least until nemesis overtakes us in the form of degenerative diseases such as arthritis, high blood-pressure, cancer, coronary heart disease and bronchitis. By comparison with these crippling and often fatal diseases, tinnitus and catarrhal deafness may, perhaps, be regarded as being relatively small penalties to pay for our ignorance and thoughtlessness, although the distress and misery which they cause is often considerable.

Fortunately, however, once their background causes are understood, much can be done gradually to reduce the severity of the symptoms and restore the delicate and very complex hearing mechanisms to a higher degree of functional efficiency.

2

Fallacies and Misconceptions

Tinnitus and catarrhal deafness are afflictions mainly of those who are already middle-aged or older. It is understandable, therefore, that sufferers will have some difficulty in discarding ideas and beliefs implanted during childhood and nurtured throughout their lifetime by a succession of 'experts' who, in the press, on radio and television, in books and magazines and through every other medium of communication, have propagated the orthodox medical conception of disease as being the result of an attack by an external agent — for example, a germ or virus — which must be fought and destroyed by the administration of potentially harmful drugs.

It is vitally important, therefore, for the reader to realize that experts are not infallible, and that many of the current views and theories which they expound so confidently will be discredited and discarded by future generations of experts, just as most of the often heroic therapeutic practices of the past are regarded today with disdain and amusement.

Especially prized among the books in my library is a well-worn copy of *Domestic Medicine* by William Buchan, MD, Fellow of the Royal College of Physicians, Edinburgh. It is dated 1800, but is the seventeenth edition of a work that was first published in 1783 — more than two hundred years ago. The author was clearly an eminent and very experienced member of his profession although he was vilified by the medical establishment, firstly for having lifted the veil of secrecy and mysticism from the practice of domestic medicine, and secondly for his insistence that in the treatment of disease too much emphasis was placed on medication and too little on what he termed 'regimen' — by which he meant diet, air, exercise, and the natural healing capacity of the human body. 'The man who pays a proper attention to these,' he wrote in the preface of his book, 'will seldom need the physician, and he who does not, will seldom enjoy health, let him employ as many physicians as he pleases.'

In those days, of course, the drug industry had not even begun to establish the massive influence over medical practice which it maintains today, and the doctor's armamentarium was confined mainly to relatively simple and harmless herbal preparations which he made up in his own pharmacy.

Dr Buchan does not hesitate to advise his readers regarding the proper use of these simple remedies, but despite his undoubted broadmindedness in many other respects he betrays the inevitable human limitations inherent in all generations of 'experts' when he pins his faith on blood-letting as the treatment of choice in a wide variety of illnesses ranging from asthma to yaws. The confidence with which he recommends this long-since abandoned therapeutic measure is mirrored today by that of the 'experts' who proclaim the 'magic' of the current miracle-drugs:

'No operation of surgery,' Dr Buchan maintained, 'is so frequently necessary as bleeding. But though practised by midwives, gardeners, blacksmiths, & c. we have reason to believe that very few know when it is proper.

'Bleeding is proper at the beginning of all fevers, in inflammations of the intestines, womb, bladder, stomach, kidneys, throat, eyes & c. and also in the asthma, sciatic pains, coughs, headaches and rheumatisms, the apoplexy, epilepsy and bloody flux. After falls, blows, bruises, or any violent hurt received either externally or internally, bleeding is necessary.'

Is it not significant that today, two hundred years after these words were written, Dr Buchan's profound observations concerning the value of diet, fresh air, exercise and the general principles of natural healing are still propagated and gaining wide public acceptance, whereas the blood-letting and other dangerous and unnatural practices which were in vogue at that time have long since been relegated to limbo, where in due course they will undoubtedly be joined by the even more potent and dangerous drugs, vaccines and 'spare-part' surgery which are the stock-in-trade of today's high priests of medicine?

We do not have to go beyond recent history to find graphic evidence of medical fallibility. For example, the thalidomide disaster is still being brought home to us through the medium of television documentaries and press reports concerning the progress and achievements of some of the grossly deformed victims who were born to women who were pregnant when their doctors prescribed the drug.

Unfortunately, it is only very rarely that harmful side-effects can be clearly attributed to a particular drug in a short period of time, and in most cases many years elapse before a drug, which will have been 'cleared' as safe and effective after extensive tests — first on laboratory animals and then on human patients — is found to cause serious systemic and organic disorders.

Aspirin

The human body has, as we have already observed, an extraordinary capacity for defence against abuse, and it will tolerate misuse for many years before signs of weakness and breakdown become apparent. An example of this is provided by aspirin which, for more than half a century, was regarded almost universally as a simple and safe panacea for a host of common ailments such as colds, influenza and headaches. Today, the medical pharmacopoeia devotes no less than three and a half closely printed pages to the toxic effects, their treatment, and the precautions to be observed when prescribing this 'harmless' remedy of which many millions of tablets annually are still being bought from chemists and supermarkets.

But for the fact that aspirin replaced cortisone — itself the cause of many serious side-effects — as the treatment of choice for arthritis it could well have been many more years before the harm it causes was recognized. There is no effective medical treatment for arthritis, and in order to afford an acceptable level of pain relief it was necessary for doctors to prescribe a relatively high dosage of aspirin to be taken almost indefinitely in many cases, as a result of which its ill-effects were eventually highlighted. The list of side-effects which became apparent in patients subjected to a sustained high dosage includes dizziness, sweating, nausea, vomiting, mental confusion and fever. Even small doses may cause gastric irritation, dyspepsia, gastric ulceration, vomiting of blood and blood-stained faeces.

Slight blood-loss, says the report, may recur in about 70 per cent of patients with most aspirin preparations, whether they are buffered, soluble or plain, but this loss, it continues reassuringly, is not usually of clinical significance, although it may cause iron-deficiency anaemia during long-term therapy.

To complete the list of side-effects — and of special interest in the context of the subject of this book — it is significant that *aspirin can also be a cause of tinnitus!* Another drug which has been similarly implicated is quinine which, in combination with other substances, may be prescribed for the relief of pain and feverish conditions.

Since tinnitus and deafness are closely associated with catarrhal congestion of the nose and throat it is also relevant to say that sprays containing drugs such as adrenaline and isoprenaline, which are prescribed as inhalants and decongestants, can also cause many harmful reactions, including anxiety, breathlessness, restlessness, pulse irregularities, tremors, weakness, dizziness, headache, vomiting, cold hands and feet, increased nasal congestion and chronic inflammation of the nasal mucous membranes.

Drug-orientated Medical Practice

Regrettable as it may seem that modern medical thinking and practice are almost entirely drug-orientated, and that the importance of diet, fresh air and exercise (stressed so emphatically by Dr Buchan two hundred years ago) is rarely if ever considered, it is easily understandable when we realize the extent to which medical training has allowed itself to be dominated by the vast international drug industry.

The training which the medical student undergoes in order to qualify for general practice is long and arduous. Initially, he has to acquire a detailed understanding of human anatomy and physiology, followed by an equally intensive study of disease signs and symptoms and the techniques of diagnosis. Somewhere along the way the effects of nutrition and environmental factors may be mentioned briefly, but throughout the course the main emphasis is on medication — what drugs must be prescribed for each specific disease entity. At the end of his training the student will graduate only if he gives the right answers to the questions set by his examiners — answers based on the knowledge instilled in him by his tutors and supported by the textbooks approved by the medical establishment. Having overcome all these daunting hurdles, he may then be required to serve an apprenticeship as a junior practitioner in a hospital where conformity with accepted medical principles will be demanded by his seniors.

After many years of constant indoctrination he will probably take his place as a fully qualified, but still very junior, member of a group of GPs caught up in a busy round of surgery sessions and house calls which leave him with little time or inclination to question the validity of what he has been taught. In the few minutes which he can allow each patient, he can only ask enough brief questions to enable him to allocate a 'label' to the patient's health problems, before reaching for his pen and scribbling a prescription for the drug of his choice.

In making that choice he will have the enthusiastic co-operation of the drug manufacturers who will subject him to a daily bombardment of generous samples of their latest, improved wonder-drugs together with masses of glossy literature extolling the virtues and therapeutic properties of their products — which are, of course, safer, speedier and more effective than anything previously available. To reinforce the postal sales campaign he may be favoured with a personal visit from a representative of the company, and, if his professional status is sufficiently high, a generous gift may be left on his desk or he may even be invited to join other influential practitioners at an expenses-paid 'conference' in some salubrious holiday resort at home or abroad where, of course, every opportunity will be taken to convince him of the virtues of his host's products.

We have dealt with this subject at some length in order to explain — though not justify — the very narrow and unimaginative approach of the average GP to the subjects of health and disease. The all-powerful chemical industry not only brainwashes him continuously with drug propaganda, but also provides generous funds for medical research projects which form the basis for the production of new wonder-drugs — to supersede earlier wonder-drugs which have failed to live up to the claims made for them or which have become unacceptable because of the side-effects which have eventually become manifest.

Supression of Symptoms
It is a sad fact that while dangerous drugs can be sold at exorbitant prices to make vast profits for the chemical industry, it is very much more difficult to package and market the therapeutic measures which alone can bring real and lasting health — i.e. simple whole foods, exercise, fresh air, sound sleep and recreation. And, human nature being what it is, the patient will always prefer to have his health problems solved for him by simply swallowing a few pills or a few doses of medicine; that is very much less demanding than being required to accept responsibility for his own body and seek

salvation by making a number of fundamental changes in the way of life to which he has become accustomed since childhood.

Unfortunately, any benefit achieved the easy way by simply suppressing unpleasant symptoms is inevitably short-lived. What he has done is akin to tightening down the safety-valve of a boiler to prevent the escape of excessive steam pressure, without reducing the heat beneath it. The pressure will continue to build up inside the boiler until it reaches a point where the steam will force its way out more fiercely than ever — either by blowing the valve or bursting the boiler.

Acute illnesses such as colds, catarrh and fevers are safety-valves which enable the body to discharge an excessive build-up of toxic waste from the tissues. If they are allowed to run their natural course recovery will be speedy and the patient will regain his full health and vitality without any untoward complications. If, however, the fever, the cough, the perspiration and the mucus discharge are suppressed with the aid of aspirin, antibiotics, or any other form of medication, the tissue poisons will be forced back into the body where they will continue to simmer for a time before breaking out again with increased virulence. In the meantime, the patient is likely to feel sluggish, tire easily and suffer from headaches, poor appetite and general malaise.

With each recurring upset the increasing burden of toxic waste will be forced deeper into the tissues and organs of the body. What may have started as a series of simple head colds will gradually extend to the throat, the sinuses, the bronchial tubes and the lungs. In the process, the Eustachian tube which connects the throat to the middle ear will become inflamed and congested, the end result of which is likely to be increasing catarrhal deafness and tinnitus.

Natural Immunity

We cannot conclude this chapter without disposing of the all-too-widely-held belief that acute flare-ups such as colds, influenza and fevers — including ear infections — are caused by germs and viruses which can attack a perfectly healthy person who has the misfortune to come into close proximity with someone who is already infected. If this theory were valid, no individual would escape from the resulting epidemic which would spread like wild-fire throughout the entire population.

It is irrefutable that certain types of germs and bacteria are present in every human. They are minute plant-like organisms so small that many thousands of them could be accommodated on the tiniest speck of dust. But far from being predators which 'attack' us and cause disease, they are in fact an essential part of the natural order of things, their function being to act as scavengers and break down complex plant and animal residues into simpler substances. Indeed, some of them exist in the digestive system where they perform a vital service by, among other things, synthesizing certain vitamins, whereas others — the so-called 'disease germs' — can only become active and proliferate in an unhealthy body which provides them with the right conditions for their survival and reproduction. These conditions do not exist in a healthy system, and so, no matter to what extent a fit person is exposed to 'infection', the germs will not be able to flourish and he will remain totally immune to infection.

On the other hand, individuals who are generally run down and in poor condition will have no such natural resistance and will readily fall victims to any infectious illness to which they may be exposed. A popular medical dictionary concedes that 'some persons expose themselves again and again to the risk of infection and are not affected, whilst others seem prone to contracting any disease with which they are brought into contact'.

The obvious inference — but one which the medical profession seems unable or unwilling to accept — is that a healthy body has the necessary degree of natural immunity which acts as an effective deterrent to harmful bacteria, and that the latter can only invade an unhealthy body which provides the sort of environment in which they can flourish and multiply. Were it not for this seemingly irrefutable fact, doctors, nurses and others who work in hospitals would succumb to recurring 'attacks' of every conceivable type of infectious illness.

Is it not more logical to assume that germs enter an already unhealthy body as scavengers, thrive for a time on the toxic debris which is the real cause of disease, and depart when the poisons on which they flourish have been flushed out of the system as a result of the greatly increased activities of the skin, bowels, kidneys and lungs which are a feature of all acute illness? When this assumption is accepted, the folly and futility of using antibiotics and other potentially harmful drugs to destroy the germs become clear.

It is analogous to reasoning that the flies which swarm around a dustbin are the cause of the foul smell emitted from the rotting refuse therein and assuming that if the flies are killed off with the aid of a poisonous insecticide spray the air will be restored to its natural sweetness. Flies, and germs, will only cease to be troublesome when the toxic debris on which they feed and flourish is destroyed.

Fortunately, there are increasing signs that the more discerning members of the public, and even a few doctors, are realizing the futility of 'fighting' disease and recognizing the fact that the only logical way to eliminate disease is to identify and remove its causes — which, in simple terms, means building health and natural immunity.

There is little doubt that the reader of this book will already have tried some of the drugs, ear-drops and other orthodox 'remedies' in an effort to rid himself of the distressing and often embarrassing symptoms of tinnitus and deafness and that he has failed to obtain any acceptable degree of lasting improvement.

It is hoped, therefore, that what he has read in the preceding pages will have helped him to understand the reasons why his own and his doctor's efforts have proved totally abortive, and encouraged him to put aside preconceived notions concerning the nature and causes of his disability. He should now be prepared to proceed, with an open and unbiased mind, to consider the alternative approach which I shall shortly be explaining.

First, however, it is necessary to show how the healthy ear should function, and what goes wrong with the delicate and extraordinarily ingenious mechanism to cause tinnitus and deafness.

3.

How the Ear Works

As is the case with many other parts of the body, the ear is very much taken for granted by most people — until, that is, something goes wrong with it. The ear is a complex mechanism by means of which the vibrations set up by the multitude of sounds generated in the immediate environment are collected and channelled through to the brain, where they are sorted and translated into meaningful messages and perhaps warnings.

For practical purposes the ear can be divided into three separate parts — the external ear, the middle ear and the inner ear (see Figure 1 on page 25).

The external and visible part, called the pinna, is shaped like a funnel and is designed so as to enable sound-waves to be collected and channelled along a tubular passage, approximately 4cm ($1\frac{1}{2}$ inches) in length. At the inner end of this tube, called the external meatus, the vibrations impinge on the ear-drum — a thin membrane which separates the external ear from the middle ear. In the middle ear are three tiny bones called the malleus (hammer), the incus (anvil) and the stapes (stirrup). These

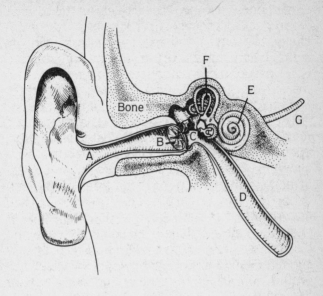

A. External Ear (Pinna)

B. Ear-drum

C. Middle Ear

D. Eustachian Tube

E. Cochlea
}
F. Semi-circular } Inner Ear
   Canals

G. Auditory Nerve

Figure 1: The hearing and balance mechanisms of the outer, middle, and inner ear chambers

three bones — known collectively as the ossicles — are linked together in that order to form a chain, the outer end of the malleus being in contact with the ear-drum, and the inner end of the stirrup being connected to another thin membrane (the oval window) which separates the middle ear from the inner chamber.

The middle ear is connected to the back of the nose and throat by the Eustachian tube, approximately 3cm (1¼ inches) in length, thus allowing the passage of air to equalize atmospheric pressure on both sides of the ear-drum. If this tube becomes narrowed or blocked as a result of catarrhal congestion the sense of hearing may be dulled to some extent, and discomfort or even pain will be caused by any sudden change in atmospheric pressure such as occurs in a lift or on take-off or landing in an aeroplane.

The inner ear houses a coiled tube — the cochlea — which is filled with fluid, the wider end of which is sealed by the oval window, while the 'tail' is connected to the brain via the auditory nerve which consists of some 30,000 or so tiny fibres. Miraculously, these tiny organs are capable of receiving and passing on to the brain a fantastic range and variety of sounds, filtering out those which are of little or no immediate concern to the recipient and sorting and classifying the relatively small number which, at any particular time, may have a bearing on his immediate needs — and even survival.

Sound

What we term 'sound' consists of vibrations

transmitted in the form of air-waves which vary in length and depth, from the very short and fast high-frequency waves corresponding to high-pitched sounds such as whistles and bird-song, to the slow, long, low-pitched sounds such as the low notes of a mighty organ or an explosion.

All these waves are collected by the shell-shaped pinna and funnelled along the external meatus to the ear-drum. The vibrations then impinge on this sensitive membrane and are relayed by the ossicles through the middle ear to the oval window which transmits them to the fluid in the coiled cochlea. It is here that the vibrations are picked up by a mass of microscopic membranes, the roots of which are connected to the thousands of nerve fibres which make up the auditory nerve, generating and transmitting to the brain nerve impulses of varying strength and frequency which are instantaneously translated by the brain to enable us to identify the source and nature of the originating sounds. This is the miracle which enables us to hear and recognize sounds as varied as a pin-drop or an entire philharmonic orchestra.

Balance

This, however, is not the only function of the ear, for tucked away in the inner ear chamber, just above the cochlea, are three U-shaped tubes known as the semi-circular canals, which are set at right-angles to each other. They are filled with fluid and act rather like a very complex set of spirit-levels so as to register body movements. One tube, set vertically, responds to up-and-down movements, another, set horizontally, records sideways movements, and the third, also horizontal but at right-angles to the second, registers fore-and-aft movements.

All this is accomplished by means of many thousands of tiny hairs, tipped with sensors, which are suspended within the semi-circular canals in such a way that when the head is moved in any direction the fluid is displaced, causing the sensors to move in sympathy. Nerve impulses are generated and transmitted from the sensors to the brain via a part of the auditory nerve. These ingenious mechanisms thus play a vital role in enabling us to maintain balance and determine the speed and direction of any bodily movement.

Disruption

Despite the care which nature has taken to protect the many delicate and complex mechanisms which are packed into such a tiny space, it is inevitable that the ear should be vulnerable to disruption from certain quarters — both external and internal.

In young children, the outer passage of the ear is quite frequently blocked because they cannot resist the temptation to push beads and other small objects into it, and even adults may misguidedly probe too deeply in an effort to dislodge an accumulation of hardened wax. Sometimes, too, a plug of cotton-wool may be inserted as a safeguard against excessive noise or to ease the pain of earache and some of the material may form a plug with hardened wax and remain lodged deep in the cavity where, in time, it can cause inflammation, infection, and, in severe cases, perforation of the ear-drum.

A severe blow on the ear or a loud explosion may generate an intense wave of air-pressure which may also rupture the ear-drum, although this type of injury to healthy tissue usually heals spontaneously and leaves no permanent impairment of hearing.

The inner ear, on the other hand, is almost totally surrounded by bony tissue and so is protected from external forces except for a blow of sufficient force to crack the skull. The auditory nerve may also be damaged by being subjected for long periods to excessive noise — a condition termed 'boiler-maker's disease'.

The delicate mechanism of the inner ear is, however, vulnerable to disruption by certain severe feverish illnesses such as mumps, meningitis and typhoid. The auditory nerve may also be temporarily affected by drugs such as quinine and aspirin.

It is the middle ear which is most frequently disrupted because, although it is not as readily accessible to harmful external factors, it has a direct connection with the nose and throat via the Eustachian tube. The nose and throat are the most common foci of catarrhal congestion and inflammation which can thus extend up the tube, restrict or even prevent the passage of air to the middle ear, or immobilize the three tiny bones which link the ear-drum with the cochlea.

Here, then, are the mechanisms which are responsible for tinnitus and catarrhal deafness: inflammation of the middle ear disrupts the operation of the ossicles, causing false impulses to be transmitted through the cochlea to the brain where they are interpreted as ringing, hissing and humming sounds, while catarrhal mucus secreted in the Eustachian tube and middle ear impairs the functional capacity of the ear-drum and the ossicles.

4.

Catarrh is the Enemy

Those readers who have observed the injunction in our first chapter and read carefully and patiently through the preceding pages will now, it is hoped, have a clear understanding of the origins of the catarrhal conditions which have disorganized the delicate mechanisms of the ear. They will also understand the complex processes on which normal sound perception is dependent and the reasons why orthodox medication can do little more than afford some temporary relief from the distressing symptoms of tinnitus and catarrhal deafness.

We can now go on to the next stage and explain why catarrh is such a widespread problem, particularly among older people, and what has gone wrong in the ear to so radically disorganize the mechanism and either prevent it from carrying out its proper functions or cause it to transmit false or distorted signals to the brain.

Causes of Tinnitus and Deafness

First, however, it is necessary to explain that there are several different causes of tinnitus and deafness, some of which can be corrected, or at least alleviated, by rational treatment methods while others, unfortunately, are likely to be irreversible. The former can be categorized, broadly, as types of *conductive* deafness, while the latter are described as forms of *perceptive* deafness.

As the terms imply, conductive deafness occurs as a result of obstruction of the airway through which the sound-waves are passed to the cochlea; it is centred, therefore, in the *outer* and *middle* chambers of the ear. Perceptive deafness, on the other hand, results from damage to or degenerative changes in the *inner* ear and the auditory nerve, thus reducing or blocking the transmission of sound impulses from the cochlea to the brain.

Testing the Degree of Deafness

Provided that only one ear is affected, there is a simple but quite effective method of differentiating between treatable obstructive deafness and irreversible perceptive deafness. It involves the use of an ordinary spring-operated watch with a clearly audible tick which is pressed against the centre of the forehead. If deafness is due to nerve damage the tick will be heard only in the good ear, but if obstruction is responsible the tick will be detected by the 'deaf' ear.

To take the self-testing process a stage further, it is possible to assess the extent to which the hearing is impaired with the aid of an assistant. The patient should sit with one ear towards the assistant, the opposite ear being closed by finger-pressure. Starting at a distance of 6 metres (approximately 20 feet), the assistant advances one pace at a time, counting slowly in a clear conversational voice, until the patient is able to hear and repeat accurately each number spoken. The criterion for assessing the degree of deafness is that in a quiet room the tester's normal conversational voice should be heard at the full distance of 6 metres.

This test affords a useful means of checking progress during the course of treatment, with the reservation, however, that in some cases of obstructive deafness — for example, where impacted wax is the cause — there may be periodic variations in hearing acuity.

For obvious reasons, I am not concerned here with the irreversible cases of perceptive deafness which have developed as a result of damage to the inner ear consequent upon head injury, high blood-pressure, anaemia, drug side-effects and prolonged exposure to excessive noise. My sole objective is to help those far more numerous victims of deafness and tinnitus resulting from catarrhal impairment of the conductive mechanisms of the outer and middle chambers of the ear.

Catarrh

Catarrh is undoubtedly one of the most widespread health problems today, and its effects are by no means confined to the nose, throat and lungs where it is universally recognized as the cause of coughs, nasal congestion, bronchitis, tonsillitis, etc. These are but the primary sites of the congestion and inflammation which, if not treated effectively, can spread to virtually all tissues and organs throughout the system, including the skin, the stomach, the bowels and colon, the liver, the eyes, the sinuses and the ears. Most of these catarrhal disorders give rise to obvious signs or symptoms of physical distress such as the stomach pains of gastric 'flu, the headache and nausea of migraine, the diarrhoea of colitis, and the inflammation of the eyes resulting from conjunctivitis.

Catarrhal deafness and tinnitus, however, present no such outward indications of the distress and disability to which they give rise, and the victim often has to bear the added stress caused by the sense of isolation and lack of sympathy and understanding among family and friends. Even the patient's GP may give the impression that the problem is a trivial one and that the sufferer should 'learn to live with it'.

At best, the ear may be syringed or a sedative drug may be prescribed, with little or no lasting benefit — for the obvious reason that the inflamed and congested mucous membranes continue their excessive secretion of mucus into the Eustachian tube and middle ear, and to exude the waxy substance which hardens and blocks the outer ear (see Figure 2, page 35).

Clearly, salvation can come only if we find and implement an effective means of (a) reducing the excessive wax secretion which blocks the outer ear and prevents the ear-drum from responding to sound waves, (b) clearing the middle ear of fluid and mucus which impedes the transmission of those vibrations to the cochlea via the malleus, incus and stapes, and

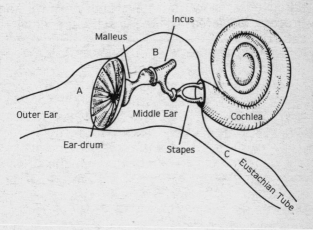

A. Wax in outer ear.

B. Fluid in middle ear.

C. Mucous secretion and swelling of Eustachian tube

Figure 2: The main causes of tinnitus and catarrhal deafness

(c) reducing the mucous secretion and swelling which block the passage of air through the Eustachian tube to the middle ear.

In other words, we must identify the causes of these distressing conditions and begin the admittedly slow but eventually rewarding process of defeating the insidious enemy — catarrh.

5.

Symptoms — Their Origin and Meaning

As I have shown in the previous chapter, tinnitus and deafness are but symptoms of a long-standing and insidious imbalance in body chemistry brought about by a variety of unnatural habit patterns which are instilled into us over the years.

In its simplest form catarrh manifests itself as the common cold which, though not usually serious, is undoubtedly one of the major causes of absence from work in the UK, particularly among the male population. Yet all the resources of the medical profession and the frenzied efforts of the drug companies to find a cure and reap the rich rewards which would undoubtedly accrue therefrom have failed totally to make any significant progress.

The Common Cold Research Unit, set up in Salisbury many years ago, pays human guinea-pigs to spend varying periods of time in conditions of carefully monitored isolation from all outside influences in the hope that, should they 'catch a cold', the scientists will be able to isolate a specific 'germ' or 'virus' and claim a resounding triumph for medical progress. Despite all the scientific and financial resources which have been harnessed to this end the Unit's efforts — and the sacrifices of the hundreds of willing guinea-pigs — have still made no headway towards the desired goal.

The GP today — like his forebears for the past half-century or more — can only advise anyone who 'catches' a cold to go to bed, keep warm, and take two aspirins every four hours or so in order to relieve the fever, sore throat, etc. If a cough develops, it is likely that a linctus containing codeine will be prescribed, or perhaps a decongestant to relieve the discomfort of blocked nostrils.

This chain of events is likely to recur at least twice a year and possibly three or even four times in a bad winter or an unusually poor summer, but the sequence may be punctuated from time to time by an attack of influenza. The symptoms on these occasions are broadly similar to those of the common cold, but they are appreciably more severe — fever, headaches, weakness, loss of appetite, generalized aches and pains throughout the body, and a feeling of depression. Again, there is no medical panacea — only aspirins to reduce the temperature and relieve the patient's general discomfort. In the more severe cases, however, antibiotics may be prescribed in order to reduce the risk of pneumonia or some other serious respiratory complication.

Over the years, this recurring sequence of events — acute feverish episodes the symptoms of which are regularly damped down and aborted by suppressive medication — causes changes to take place in the much-abused mucous membranes which line the air passages. They become thickened and increasingly fibrous, and the mucous secretions lose their thin, watery consistency and become tough and glutinous; the condition is now classified as chronic catarrh.

At this stage there can be a variety of other symptoms, the nature and severity of which can vary widely from one individual to another depending upon the susceptibility of the organs and tissues and their strengths and weaknesses as predetermined by hereditary and genetic factors.

Among the more common catarrhal afflictions are a profuse discharge of mucus from the nose; a persistent cough producing varying amounts of stringy mucus; watering eyes; sore throat; mouth-breathing and snoring at night; recurring bouts of sneezing; sinusitis; swollen glands; dandruff and thinning hair; and, of course, tinnitus and deafness. It is probable that only an infinitely small proportion of the population of the UK remains free from one or other of these conditions throughout the year, and it is claimed in an authoritative report that there are some eight million people in this country who suffer to some extent from tinnitus alone.

Poor Diet

Clearly, what is virtually a universal problem must have an equally universal cause, and I have no hesitation in asserting that the conventional diet must take the major share of the blame.

We have only to wander around any

supermarket and note what goes into the trolleys to realize that probably 90 per cent of the average purchases consist of canned, bottled, packaged and preserved produce which has been processed, chemicalized and denatured to such an extent that it bears little or no resemblance to the natural product from which it may have originated.

White flour has been refined, bleached and deprived of virtually all nutritive value, and has then been 'fortified' with synthetic chemical substances in order to restore some semblance of pseudo food value.

White sugar has suffered even more at the hands of the processors, and the end-product — purchased and consumed in vast quantities in this country — fulfils no physiological function which cannot be performed far more effectively and safely by other foods.

To quote from a standard nutritional reference book, *Human Nutrition and Dietetics*, by Sir Stanley Davidson and R. Passmore: 'As a cheap and easily digested form of energy, sugar is a valuable food; but as it lacks every nutrient save carbohydrate, its very attractiveness is a danger in that it tends to displace more nutritious food from the diet. Coincident with the increase in the sugar consumption there was an increase in the incidence of dental disease.

'Chemists have devoted much technical ingenuity to removing the last traces of 'impurities' from commercial sucrose... Crystalline table sugar is thus one of the purest chemicals regularly produced in large quantities by modern industry. It is practically 100 per cent sucrose and contains no other nutrients, such as minerals and vitamins.'

Apart from its destructive effect on teeth — and even children are now having to be fitted with dentures — there is sound evidence to link the ever-rising consumption of sugar with a parallel increase in the incidence of coronary heart disease and diabetes.

Yet these two worthless commodities — white flour and white sugar — form the basis or are a substantial ingredient of many of the commercial products which fill the supermarket shelves, most of them being laced in addition with a wide range of chemicals in the form of colourings, preservatives, flavourings and texturizers. As a not untypical example, the package containing a popular 'dessert-whip' mixture lists the following ingredients: Sugar, modified starch (E1404), acidity regulators (E450a, E341a, E341b), salt, flavouring, colours (E102, E110, Brown HT, E142, E123).

Beneath this catalogue of chemical concoctions the manufacturers add a 'guarantee' to the effect that they promise to refund your money if you are not entirely satisfied with either the high quality or value for money of this item.

One can only marvel at the naïvety of a 'food' producer who can describe such a product as being either high quality or value for money!

I have said in an earlier chapter that the human body has an extraordinary capacity for adaptation and compensation, and that it strives continually to maintain the functional efficiency of its organs and tissues no matter to what extent it is abused and misused. The fact remains, however, that to a large extent man is what he eats, and there must come a time when tissues which have been consistently poisoned and deprived of essential nutrients will begin to break down under the strain.

Defence Mechanisms

The body's first lines of defence against nutritional abuse are the eliminative organs — the bowels, the kidneys and the skin — through which are excreted the unwanted residues of food solids and liquids. Under severe stress, they will react to the emergency by initiating vomiting, diarrhoea and feverish perspiration in order to rid the body quickly of an overload of potentially harmful substances. These dramatic protective reactions are, however, usually activated only when the organism is put under immediate threat, such as when tainted food or water is taken, or when a large quantity of alcohol or a drug has been consumed. In these situations, the body's defence mechanisms are immediately brought into play, the offending substances are ejected, and normal systemic equilibrium is usually restored within twenty-four hours or so.

A different situation arises, however, when the body is subjected daily to an insidious infiltration of relatively small doses of chemicals and other harmful substances and/or is persistently deprived of essential nutrients — vitamins, minerals, fibre, amino acids or any of the myriad other constituents needed for tissue repair, maintenance and growth.

It is in an effort to cope with this all-too-common situation that the body calls upon its extensive powers of adaptation and compensation in an effort to make the best of the available resources and neutralize those alien substances which threaten to disrupt the complex biochemical functions of the digestive system, the liver and the glandular system.

'Complex' is, in fact, an all-too-inadequate term to describe human biochemistry.

Thanks to the efforts of popular journalists and television programme producers, most of us are now reasonably familiar with the basic functions of our bodies. Few people can now be ignorant of the fact that overeating causes obesity and that starchy and sugary foods are the main culprits in this respect. We are reminded frequently that salt has been indicated as a contributory causative factor in high blood-pressure, that cigarette smoking increases substantially one's liability to contract cancer of the throat and lungs, that over-indulgence in alcohol leads to liver failure, and that too much sugar in the diet increases the risk of coronary heart disease.

But medical research still stubbornly refuses to accept the possibility that faulty nutrition is the key factor in virtually all the acute illnesses, and it is because of this extraordinary blind spot that the incidence of chronic disease is continually increasing and that relatively young people are succumbing to illnesses which not so many years ago were afflicting only the elderly.

No one would deny the assertion that a

first-class product can only be produced from carefully selected materials of the highest quality, and yet the human body is expected to maintain itself and continue to function efficiently on a hotch-potch of manufactured, manipulated and denatured products which do not bear the slightest resemblance to the raw materials — the natural whole foods — which nature provided for our use.

A skilled chemist knows that, when working in his laboratory, he must adhere meticulously to a precise formula in order to produce a consistent end-product. The slightest deviation can cause an unwanted reaction and wreck an important experiment.

The human body functions and maintains itself by means of a continuous interaction of minerals, vitamins, enzymes and other elements which it can obtain only from the food we eat, the liquids we drink and the air we breath. We are all only too well aware that if the body is totally deprived of any of these vital substances death is inevitable — very speedily when the air supply is cut off, and more slowly when water or food is withheld.

Is it not entirely logical, therefore, to expect that some degree of breakdown or malfunction will occur if the body is deprived of the right materials needed for its maintenance and repair, and if its complex biochemical processes are disrupted by the ingestion of the myriads of extraneous chemical substances which are listed on the labels of virtually every can, package and bottle to be found on the supermarket shelves?

The Lymphatic System

We have said that the bowels, kidneys and skin are the body's first line of defence against nutritional abuse, but far more subtle is the role of the lymphatic system, the protective functions of which are rarely mentioned by the popular media and of which most people are totally unaware.

Lymph is a thin, colourless fluid, its constitution being very much akin to that of blood plasma, from which it is derived. As blood circulates throughout the body some of its watery constituents pass through the walls of the capillaries into the tissues, carrying nutrients to the body cells and absorbing waste products. It is then collected by lymph capillaries which unite to form tiny vessels like minute veins which gradually coalesce to form larger ducts which eventually empty their contents into the large veins at the base of the neck.

At various strategic points — behind the knee, in the groin, in the neck and the armpits — the lymphatic system is punctuated by groups of lymph nodes or glands containing specialized white blood corpuscles, the function of which is to filter out, neutralize and destroy toxic substances, bacteria and other potentially harmful materials and thus prevent them from entering the bloodstream.

The lymph vessels, like the veins, do not benefit from the pumping action of the heart which propels the blood through the arteries, but depend instead upon the contraction and relaxation of adjacent muscles to force the lymph upwards, assisted by a series of valves which prevent any backflow.

This brief description underlines the importance of the lymphatic system in the body's defences and explains why, when the tissues become overloaded with toxic substances and cell wastes, the glands become hard and enlarged. Examples which will be familiar to many people are the swollen glands beneath the angle of the jaw which become readily palpable when we suffer from tonsillitis or a sore throat, and a similar swelling in the armpit if a boil erupts in the vicinity.

This also emphasizes the importance of regular physical exercise as a means of promoting bodily health, since the sluggish circulation of blood and lymph which results from habitual inactivity both starves the tissues of blood-born oxygen and nutrients and seriously hampers the body's cleansing and protective functions.

It is to a large extent the combination of faulty nutrition and physical inactivity which allows toxic material to accumulate in the tissues, causing them to become increasingly inflamed and congested, thus explaining why our failure to deal effectively with minor colds and catarrh leads eventually to more deep-seated problems such as tinnitus and catarrhal deafness.

These are important factors which the sufferer must understand clearly in order to appreciate the simple logic of the various treatment measures which must be undertaken in order not merely to obtain some measure of relief from distressing symptoms but — what is even more desirable — to achieve a much greater degree of freedom from the fear of recurring and worsening attacks of these and other catarrhal afflictions.

It cannot be stressed too strongly or too frequently that the aim of natural, drugless healing is not merely the relief of any specific group of symptoms, no matter what label may be attached to them, but the restoration of total health. That, surely, is a consummation devoutly to be wished!

6.

The Natural Approach

The first and most fundamental principle of natural healing is that the body must be allowed to carry out its own curative and restorative functions. No illness can be 'cured' by any external agency, whether it be in the form of medicine, surgery, spiritual healing, hypnotism, manipulation, acupuncture, radiation or any other specific treatment.

Over the years there has been a continuing search for the 'magic elixir' which will 'cure' the many and various diseases and disabilities to which human flesh is heir, but no sooner do we appear to have eliminated one particular scourge than another takes its place and the search for a new magic remedy starts all over again. It can be asserted with complete confidence that no matter how many millions of pounds are spent on medical research, we shall still be enduring a similar, if not greater, burden of illness in fifty or a hundred years' time unless there is a radical change in medical thought and practice.

Fortunately, there are signs that disillusionment — and enlightenment — is already quite widespread in the minds of the lay public, who are increasingly turning away from the traditional pills and potions and seeking a solution to their health problems from the ranks of what has come to be termed 'alternative medicine'. This is a very encouraging trend, but all too often those who take this new path do so in the hope and belief that they can be cured simply by substituting a simple 'natural' remedy for the potent and harmful drugs on which they have relied in the past. Inevitably, their hopes will be dashed, for the simple reason that the only source of a really lasting cure lies within the ailing body itself — by releasing and mobilizing the vital resources which alone can eliminate tissue poisons, renew damaged tissues and restore functional efficiency to impaired organs.

The vital power which can accomplish this transformation is the same power which keeps the heart beating day after day, year after year, throughout our lives; which renews the skin that protects our bodies; which enables us to see, hear and feel; which takes complex minerals and other substances from our food and utilizes them to replace worn-out tissues and to maintain and stabilize body heat.

These are but a few of the miracles which are being accomplished continuously and unobtrusively every day of our lives and which we take so much for granted.

Surely, then, it is logical to assume that this same vital power, which can repair broken bones and heal torn flesh without outside help, will be quite capable of carrying out essential repairs and maintenance work on any other impaired tissues and organs — if it is allowed to do so and is given the right kind of care and assistance, and the necessary raw materials.

But therein lies the rub: we do not give our bodies the right kind of care, nor do we provide it with the proper raw materials, and that is why so many things can eventually go wrong.

The food we eat is processed, chemicalized and cooked until it is virtually devoid of all nutritive value. Vitamins are destroyed by heating, exposure to air and sunlight, and overlong storage; minerals are dissolved out into the water in which our food is cooked and are then poured down the sink; important elements are removed during the refining and manufacturing processes. As if all this were not enough, the pathetic residues of what were once nutritious staple foods are coloured, flavoured and preserved with a variety of chemicals which would normally have no place in the nutritional order of things, and many of which are banned as being a health hazard by food authorities in more enlightened countries. The final insult comes when synthetic 'vitamins', produced by the chemical laboratories, are added to these 'foods' to enable the manufacturers to make spurious claims in regard to their nutritive value.

Natural Healing
Here, then, is the fundamental tenet of natural healing: The human body can and will maintain all its functions and tissues in perfect working order if it is provided with the necessary raw materials and given the necessary care and attention. It also has the capacity to repair

damaged tissues and revitalize weakened organs once we stop harming and abusing them.

Many of the symptoms of acute illness are no more than the outward manifestations of the body's desperate efforts to maintain some semblance of metabolic equilibrium in the face of continuing nutritional abuse and deprivation. In its struggle to achieve this, it mobilizes all the reserves of its eliminative organs: the body temperature is raised to induce profuse perspiration; the digestive system is cleared of unwanted food by means of vomiting and diarrhoea; the urine will become abnormally profuse and concentrated; the skin will erupt with a variety of weeping and discharging sores, boils and rashes; and the mucous membranes will produce a copious secretion of mucus.

Instead of suppressing all these self-cleansing processes, the logical procedure is to allow them to run their natural course and fulfil their allotted function — a process which in most cases will be carried out speedily and efficiently within a week or two.

To facilitate the cleansing process and so hasten recovery it is necessary merely to follow a course which is clearly signposted by the instinctive reactions of the patient:

1. *Complete rest.* The patient invariably feels weak and tired, so he should be encouraged to go to bed and sleep soundly for as long as he desires. His head and eyes will ache, so the room should be darkened.

2. *Fasting.* Even if there is no nausea or sickness, there will almost certainly be a

complete lack of appetite, so abstinence from solid food will allow the digestive system to be cleared of unwanted food residues, and vital energy will be released for more important functions.

3. *Fever.* The internal heat generated by fever and the resultant profuse perspiration will have a reflex chilling effect on the surface tissues and may even induce shivering, so that warmth must be maintained by the use of appropriate bed-covers. The bedroom should be adequately heated but good ventilation should be maintained by leaving a door or window partially open.

4. *Drinking.* The loss of body fluid through the skin, bowels and bladder will create abnormal thirst which should be satisfied by taking frequent drinks of cold water or dilute fruit or vegetable juices. Sweetened cordials and proprietary fruit drinks should not be taken, nor should milk.

5. *Bathing.* To cool the skin and remove the toxic substances excreted in the perspiration the body should be sponged periodically with cool water, and pyjamas, sheets, etc. should be changed when necessary.

The reader will, I think, have little difficulty in accepting the fact that all of these procedures conform to the dictates of natural instinct, and yet, although man is considered to be far and away the most intelligent of earthly creatures, he is in fact the only one which deliberately flouts natural dictates. One has only to observe the reactions of all kinds of domestic animals to appreciate the remarkable uniformity of their response to injuries or illness.

Faced with any such crisis, the instinct for self-preservation immediately asserts itself. They stop eating, and no matter how much we may try to tempt them with any kind of delicacy they steadfastly refuse to take anything but occasional drinks of cooling water. They seek out a quiet, dark corner and sleep soundly for hours on end, continuing to do so until well on the way to full recovery from whatever injury or illness has befallen them. Only then will they begin to take food and become progressively more active.

'Dumb' animals *know* what needs to be done under these circumstances and refuse to be diverted from the course along which they are directed by their instincts. Only intelligent man allows himself to be persuaded to ignore clear directions provided by Nature and 'feed to keep up his strength', take poisonous drugs which can only harm an already weakened system, and generally follow the misguided dictates of custom and tradition.

Then, when he finally succeeds in damping down the fire which Nature had intended should rid his body of an excess of toxic refuse, he returns to the same ill-chosen diet and other debilitating habits of living which had originally triggered off the acute illness. What should have been a cleansing and revitalizing process has been totally frustrated, and the body is left weakened and debilitated.

It is my intention in this book to explain what

needs to be done in order to harness, instead of frustrating, the vital forces with which Nature has endowed our bodies, so that not only shall we find a lasting solution to the problems of tinnitus and catarrhal deafness, but also build the solid foundation of healthy tissue and organic efficiency which alone can establish a high degree of natural immunity to all the other acute diseases which blight the lives of so many of us today.

7

A Plan of Campaign: Elimination

In the previous chapters we have explained the catarrhal origins of tinnitus and deafness, cleared away some of the more deeply ingrained prejudices and misconceptions regarding the fallaceous germ theory of disease, exposed the futility and dangers of orthodox medical treatment, and outlined the inner workings of the ear and the various types of deafness and their main causes. We have stressed the futility of suppressing symptoms and explained briefly the alternative approach which harnesses the body's innate recuperative powers based on natural but long-suppressed instincts.

Now, we can go a stage further and develop a detailed plan of action, in which we shall consciously and deliberately induce the natural tissue-cleansing processes which, had they been allowed to do so, would long since have spring-cleaned the catarrhal clutter from our tissues and restored the normal condition of physical and mental well-being which is true health.

In order to allow the body to concentrate all its vital resources on the self-curative tasks which we shall seek to set in motion, it is desirable that the treatment plan should be commenced at a time when the maximum possible degree of rest and relaxation can be assured. The ideal would be to arrange one's affairs so that for three or four days at least — and preferably for a week or more — demands on one's physical and mental resources can be kept to an absolute minimum.

For old, retired people this should present few problems, particularly if the full co-operation of a husband or wife can be enlisted, but even those who do not have the benefit of such freedom from family or business commitments may be able to arrange their affairs so that they can have a weekend or a few days' holiday during which they can take a little time off from their more demanding responsibilities, rest from time to time during the day and go to bed earlier than usual to ensure eight hours or more of sound sleep.

To appreciate the reason for these precautions it must be remembered that tinnitus and catarrhal deafness are *chronic* disorders which have developed as a result of the suppression of earlier *acute* illnesses.

The Healing Crisis

In order to enable the body to rid itself of the deep-seated toxic residues which have accumulated in the tissues — possibly over a period of many years — we shall be adopting measures which may induce the heightened eliminative responses which characterize acute disease. The speed and effectiveness of these reactions will vary from one patient to another, depending upon many factors — for example, age, general vitality, duration and extent of the ear trouble, and whether the subject is overweight or underweight.

In some cases there may be only very minor reactions such as a slight cough or cold, or a mild headache and feeling of malaise, while others — particularly the younger and more physically active types whose weight varies little from the normal for their height and physique — may react very quickly and dramatically with a raised temperature, profuse perspiration, increased mucus secretion, loss of appetite, sore throat, enlarged glands and all the other symptoms of acute illness. Any such reactions should, however, be welcomed as an indication that the body has begun the task of cleansing its tissues which it is our purpose to encourage and facilitate.

We have induced what is termed 'a healing crisis', a process of heightened elimination of accumulated toxic residues from the bloodstream as a preliminary to rebuilding the impaired organs and restoring their functional efficiency.

The onset of a healing crisis of this kind is, in fact, a clear indication that, no matter what abuse and maltreatment it may have been subjected to over the years, the body has still the vitality and the innate capacity for self-preservation which are inherent in all living creatures and which are now being mobilized and put to constructive use. It is essential that this vitally important point should be stressed at this stage so that if any such reaction should occur at any time it will not be misinterpreted and cause alarm or despondency. As we have already indicated, it should be welcomed as marking an important milestone on the road to recovery.

Understanding the Treatment

The need for a clear understanding of this phenomenon is probably greatest when well-meaning friends and relatives express concern at what appears to them to be a 'flare-up' or worsening of one's condition when, not unnaturally, they feel that there should be a steady and uninterrupted improvement if these rather strange new treatment measures are really working.

These people are, of course, conditioned by accustomed practice to be afraid of any new symptom and to regard with suspicion any unusual method of treatment, but their understandable anxiety can easily undermine one's confidence and sow seeds of doubt concerning the wisdom of continuing along the road to recovery.

Rather should one be encouraged to go forward, confident in the understanding that what is happening is in fact a clear indication that vital reserves are being mobilized on one's behalf.

With this injunction clearly in mind, we come to what is perhaps the most effective single therapeutic measure in the naturopathic armamentarium — *fasting*.

Fasting

Fasting is the most widely misunderstood and,

by the uninformed, feared procedure, because from infancy onwards it is instilled into us that we *must* eat to live and to keep up our strength. The 'three good meals a day' mentality is perhaps less widespread than it was in the past, but the ritual of eating regularly at fixed times every day is still very deeply ingrained in the vast majority of people, at least in European communities. It is, therefore, regarded as unthinkable that anyone should voluntarily forgo food for even one day, and the direst consequences are predicted if such abstinence is continued for two or even three days. And yet millions of people throughout the world regularly fast as a part of their religious observances, and consider themselves purified and uplifted as a consequence, while Nature Cure pioneers in this country (for example the late Stanley Lief and James C. Thomson) conducted therapeutic fasts of up to forty days when treating seriously ill patients in residential clinics such as Champneys, Tring, Herts. and the Kingston Clinic in Edinburgh. One such patient — the Revd Walter Wynn — published a book entitled *How I Cured Myself by Fasting* which chronicled his return to health after undergoing a fast of that duration.

Certainly, it would be very unwise for anyone to attempt any such protracted treatment without the very closest professional supervision, but with very few exceptions — notably when the patient is already extremely weak and emaciated — nothing but good can come from a short fast conducted with reasonable care by someone who has confidence in what he is doing and is not plagued by ill-founded doubts and fears. Indeed, such a relatively simple exercise in self-discipline will not only bring health benefits but afford also a not inconsiderable sense of achievement and mental satisfaction.

For the sufferer from any catarrhal trouble the short fast is undoubtedly the single most effective means of initiating the tissue-cleansing processes which must be set in motion if the troublesome inflammation and congestion are to be reduced and eventually cleared.

Since faulty nutrition is the major causative factor in all of these conditions, it is only by cutting off the intake of food for a time that the body can be given an opportunity to clear away the harmful debris as a preliminary to neutralizing and eliminating the toxic substances which have accumulated over the years in the deeper tissues of the body. All the time we continue to eat — no matter how small the quantity — the body must continue to carry out the complex chemical processes of digestion and assimilation. Once food is withheld, however, these functions are halted and the body is able to concentrate all its energies on the process of elimination. That is why fasting as a therapeutic measure is so highly valued in natural healing circles and why it is employed as a preliminary in the treatment of so many acute and chronic ailments.

In general terms, it may be claimed that a clean body, internally, is a healthy body and, conversely, an unclean body will inevitably succumb sooner or later to disease and degeneration.

In order to allay any lingering doubt concerning the safety and advisability of fasting, it is necessary, at this stage, to explain the fundamental differences between fasting and starvation — a distinction which is very widely misunderstood and often misrepresented by orthodox doctors.

Thanks to the services of newspapers, television, radio and other news agencies, most of us today are all too painfully aware of the plight of thousands — even millions — of inhabitants of famine-afflicted Third World countries who are suffering and dying as a result of widespread food shortages due to drought conditions and consequent crop failure. What we have seen is the true picture of starvation — sunken cheeks, staring eyes, distended and fluid-filled abdomen, emaciated arms and legs, protruding ribs and shoulder-blades, and an all-pervading air of apathy and despair.

By no stretch of imagination could any of these symptoms of malnutrition be related to the effects of a short fast under carefully controlled conditions. Most, if not all, of the disorders for which fasting is prescribed originate to a large extent from over-nutrition rather than under-nutrition, and when food is withheld for a relatively short time it is the surplus fatty tissue built up as a result of overeating that is drawn upon by the body in order to sustain its vital processes.

If there is any degree of obesity some of the surplus weight will undoubtedly be shed during the course of a fast, but any such loss will be minimal in a normal person unless the fasting process is extended for any reason.

It is understandable, however, that because of the lifelong habit of feeding at regular times throughout the day, the body's built-in 'time-clock' will transmit the customary hunger alarm signals at meal-times during the first day or two, but if these demands are ignored, or allayed by taking a drink of water or fruit juice, the appetite subsides very quickly. The process can be aided further by occupying one's mind by reading, watching a television programme, solving a crossword puzzle or some similar mental diversion, or simply closing one's eyes and resting or sleeping.

The signs that the cleansing processes have begun to operate will usually become apparent within 24 hours or so of the commencement of the fast. They will vary to some extent depending upon the age of the patient, his general state of health, the severity and duration of the condition for which he is being treated, whether or not he is overweight, and various other factors.

Many patients find to their surprise that far from feeling weak and listless, they actually experience an unaccustomed surge of energy and vitality and a desire to be out and about — walking, gardening or engaging in some other physical activity. Any such urge can be indulged quite safely provided that reasonable discretion is observed and the body is not subjected to any excessive or unaccustomed strain.

Towards the end of the first 24 hours it is likely that these feelings of euphoria will gradually diminish, to be replaced by some degree of lassitude. By this time, the release of toxic waste from the tissues will have begun to take effect, and as the circulation takes up this unaccustomed burden other symptoms will arise such as a headache, a furred tongue, a feeling of heaviness over the eyes, the urine will become darker and there may even be an occasional sensation of heart palpitation.

Usually, after the first day or so, the body accepts the fact that food will not be forthcoming at the usual times and appetite subsides. Coincidentally, there is likely to be an increased desire for liquids, which should be satisfied 'on demand' by drinks of water or dilute vegetable juices, thus meeting the body's need for additional fluid to act as a solvent for the toxins which are being released into the bloodstream.

In most cases the eliminative activities will have peaked by the end of the third day, and unless a healing crisis has intervened it will be time to break the fast very gradually, first by introducing small quantities of fresh fruit for a day or two and then progressively increasing and varying the food intake, but ensuring that only small meals of simple wholefoods are taken. In this way the body's digestive and assimilative systems are allowed to return gradually to their normal functional capacity, cleansed and refreshed and able to take up and utilize essential nutrients while continuing the process of elimination.

Thus the first and hardest phase of the treatment plan is completed, and we can now go on to explain the role of balanced nutrition as a means of revitalizing and rebuilding impaired tissues — a role which must be clearly understood and implemented if we are to benefit to the fullest possible extent from the efforts we have made already.

8.

The Second Phase: Rebuilding

In the preceding chapters we have stressed repeatedly that a balanced diet of simple whole foods, providing the body with the vitamins, proteins, minerals, fibre and other essential nutrients, is the foundation upon which a healthy and efficient organism is very largely dependent, and that, conversely, poor health and physical degeneration are the inevitable end-products of a diet which consists mainly of commercially processed, refined and denatured produce.

It is a subject of such far-reaching importance that we make no apology for reiterating the fundamental tenet of natural healing and healthy living that what we eat determines how our bodies will develop and function. This basic truth — that we should eat in order that we may live — has been lost sight of almost entirely in industrial societies, and instead of choosing food on the basis of its nutritional value most people today select it solely on the basis of its sensory appeal and the ease with which it can be prepared and served.

These people have long since lost sight of the fact — if they were ever aware of it — that eating is as vital a function as breathing, and instead they regard mealtimes merely as occasions when their distorted appetites can be appeased. The overriding criteria in their choice of food products are that the colour and shape of the package should appeal to the eye, that the taste of the contents should satisfy the palate, and that the product can be made ready to eat with the minimum expenditure of time and effort, and the manufacturers vie with each other in their efforts to outdo their competitors in the market place in these fields of endeavour.

Commercial considerations have gradually and increasingly replaced nutritional values not only in the food factories but even in the farming community where greater yields are forced from the soil as a result of the use of chemical fertilizers on a massive scale. Simultaneously, battery methods have been introduced which, in order to maximize the production of eggs, poultry, pork and veal, require animals and birds to be herded and confined in grossly over-crowded conditions, fed and fattened on artificially manipulated foodstuffs and doctored with hormones and antibiotics in an effort to ward off disease and stimulate rapid growth.

It is true that in recent years public opinion has brought the beginnings of a backlash against these methods, but Parliament, bowing to pressure from commercial interests and backed by its blinkered scientific and medical advisors, has refused to recognize the shortcomings of the vast bulk of the nation's food and the need for stricter quality controls and higher nutritional standards. For far too long the food industry has been encouraged to concentrate on quantity at the expense of quality. Calorie values have taken precedence over nutritional values, and we have the extraordinary situation in which invalids and children can be urged to eat and drink concoctions of sugar and chemicals by means of advertising campaigns which imply that these products hasten recovery from illness and provide abundant energy.

The medical profession, which should fulfil the role of guardians of the nation's health, see nothing wrong in all this, nor do they even concede that the food we eat is in any way responsible for much of the illness which afflicts us. It would indeed be a rarity for any GP to suggest to a patient that his badly chosen diet was largely responsible for the fact that he was suffering from tinnitus or deafness, bronchitis or asthma, tonsillitis or sinusitis. Only recently and grudgingly have they recognized that refined white flour and its products are largely responsible for constipation, colitis, diverticulitis and various other bowel disorders — a 'discovery' which they have made more than half a century after the Nature Cure pioneers first mooted the idea shortly after the First World War. Until this great breakthrough occurred in medical thinking patients suffering from these bowel troubles were actually advised to avoid wholegrain cereals, raw fruits and vegetables, and to have a 'bland diet' consisting of the very foods which are at long last being condemned.

Here again, however, the medical profession

continues to remain oblivious of the fact that it is the *quality* of our food that determines the quality of our health. Having at last recognized that the removal of bran from flour during the milling process causes a number of bowel disorders they do not reach the logical conclusion that these problems will be solved if unrefined wholewheat flour is substituted for the refined product. Instead, they are content to advise the patient to buy a packet of the bran that has been removed from the flour by the millers and take it to supplement their deficient diet, just as they support the procedure of putting chalk, synthetic vitamins and iron into white flour to replace the natural nutrients which have been extracted from it.

They are incapable of understanding that a whole food containing natural nutrients in balanced quantities and combinations is a vastly different commodity from a denatured product which has been artificially 'fortified' with synthetic laboratory products.

Natural, unspoilt food as it comes from a plant or tree grown on soil that has not been poisoned with chemical fertilizers and pesticides contains all the elements in the proper proportions required by the body for the maintenance, growth and repair of all the body's tissues and the efficient functioning of all its complex systems. That is why, after the completion of a period of therapeutic fasting, it is essential that a sensible dietary régime be adopted if we are to provide the nutrients — the building materials — which alone can carry on the cleansing and curative procedures which we have set in motion. Just as sound dietetic treatment is an essential component of any natural therapeutic programme, so it is equally important to nourish the body subsequently by continuing to provide it with wholesome, natural foods.

Adopting a New Diet

Having, therefore, cleared the tissues of toxic residues by fasting, followed by a period of restrictive dieting consisting of small quantities of vitamin-rich fruits, the next stage is to increase gradually the variety and quantity of the same kind of foods with the objective of allowing the digestive system to adapt slowly to the task of dealing with new and unaccustomed nutritional problems.

For a further week or so the diet will still consist mainly of fruit but in addition to raw apples, oranges, pears, grapes, etc. it is permissible to have baked, steamed or stewed fruit, sweetened with a little honey, together with two or three tablespoons of natural, unflavoured yogurt. A daily small, mixed salad meal is also introduced.

The yogurt serves several valuable nutritional purposes at this stage of the treatment programme. Firstly, it provides a small but easily digested source of protein and calcium, but, unlike the fresh milk from which it is derived, it has been modified by a fermentation process and does not induce catarrh; also, it has a mild laxative effect, thus helping to clear the digestive tract of any toxic residues which may remain following the fasting procedure. What is even more important, however, is the fact that natural yogurt — as distinct from some of the coloured and flavoured commercial products — restores to the digestive tract beneficial bacteria which inhibit the growth of harmful bacilli and also perform a valuable service in the processes of digestion and assimilation.

The emphasis on fruit and salads as the main dietary components at this stage is important because they are a valuable source of vitamins and minerals as well as the natural fibre which is so important in promoting normal bowel function. Therefore, in addition to their nutritional value, these fresh, raw foods supplement the cleansing procedures initiated by the short fast.

It should be remembered that catarrhal conditions such as tinnitus and deafness tend to develop as a result of an abnormally high level of acidity due to an excessive consumption of acid-forming foods, especially the refined starches and sugars. Our first priority, therefore, must be to restore normal biochemical balance by increasing the consumption of those foods the digestion of which produces an alkaline reaction in the blood and other tissue fluids. Fruit and vegetables have this valuable property, provided that they are not overcooked and that sugar and salt are not added during preparation.

The aim throughout the cleansing period should be to have frequent small meals which are eaten slowly and masticated thoroughly, thus ensuring that the digestive tract will be given every opportunity to carry out fully and efficiently the complex processes of digestion and assimilation. Once this transitionary process has been completed the next stage is to further amplify the diet and establish a balanced regimen which will provide all the nutritional components required to restore and maintain all the body's tissues and functions.

We have already referred to the alkalizing effect of the cleansing diet, but to avoid misunderstanding it needs to be explained that what are sometimes referred to as 'acid fruits' have an alkaline reaction when subjected to the processes of digestion.

Individual nutritional requirements vary very widely from one individual to another — and, indeed, in the same person from one day to the next — depending upon such diverse factors as physical characteristics, changes in temperature and weather, energy expenditure and age. All of these variables interact to alter the body's need for the different types of food, and so when we attempt to set out a basic dietary plan we can do so only in the most general terms.

There is little doubt, however, that the vast majority of people living in Western countries regularly consume substantially more food than is required by the body to maintain its tissues and functions. That is a *quantitative* error which is, however, compounded by the fact that their normal diet contains far too large a proportion of the high-calorie, acid-forming foods and insufficient of the vitamin- and mineral-rich fruits and vegetables which have alkalizing properties.

It is, of course, invidious to generalize when attempting to assess individual or 'average' feeding habits, but there is little doubt that a typical day's meals in many Western communities would vary little from the following pattern, at least so far as nutritional content is concerned.

Breakfast: A cereal such as corn- or wheat-flakes either ready sweetened or served with sugar and with milk added, followed by white bread or toast and marmalade; or beans on toast, or spaghetti on toast; or an egg, or bacon, or sausage (or all three) with perhaps fried bread and followed again by bread and marmalade.

Lunch or dinner: Fish and chips (the most popular English meal according to a national public opinion poll); or hamburger and chips; or meat with boiled vegetables; followed by ice-cream or a pudding or pastry with custard, or sweetened stewed or tinned fruit with custard or ice-cream or a proprietary 'dessert mix' of uncertain origins.

Third meal: Sandwiches of white bread filled with cheese or meat or tinned fish; or cold meat or an egg with white bread or toast; or beans on toast, followed perhaps by white bread and jam or a cake or pastry.

Breakfast and the third meal will usually be accompanied by at least two cups of tea or coffee, and another cup may be taken after the main meal of the day, not to mention morning and afternoon tea and coffee breaks.

In this gastronomic scheme of things fresh fruit and salads either have no place at all or are taken as incidental extras — a sort of side-line to a sandwich lunch or a cold meat snack.

It is not difficult to see, therefore, that by the time most of this food reaches its consumer it has been virtually denuded of any vitamins it may have had in its original state, while much of its mineral content will have been similarly lost along the way. Coupled with this nutritional bankruptcy we have to recognize the appalling imbalance in regard to other less important, and even harmful, food substances which make up the bulk of these meals. Carbohydrate in the form of white bread, breakfast cereals, pasta, cakes, pastries, potatoes, jam and marmalade, honey, sugar, ice-cream and cereal-based desserts plays a prominent role in virtually every meal, as does fat in the form of cooking oil, butter, margarine, milk, cheese, eggs and meat. Salt and sugar are added freely to many dishes, in addition to the quantities which are listed on the labels of most commercial food products.

Here, then, are the basic problems which we are endeavouring to solve: Too much food, but grossly inadequate nutritional value. If we have stressed these points *ad nauseum* throughout the preceding chapters it is in order to open the reader's eyes to the abuse to which he may have unwittingly subjected his body and which has been largely responsible for much of the ill health which causes distress and misery to so many of us. It is our hope that with the clear realization of the causes of these problems will come the incentive which is needed to make changes and cultivate new habits in place of those which have become firmly entrenched over the years.

Given a sufficiently strong incentive, and the necessary will-power, changes *can* be made and old, bad habits *can* be broken and replaced by new ones. Patience and perseverance will be called for during the early stages, but the tasks become progressively less demanding with each week that passes and as the health benefits become increasingly apparent.

Tastes in food are largely acquired in early life in response to national customs, family influences and even religious taboos. What is eaten and enjoyed by the people of one country may be regarded with abhorrence by relatively close neighbours across state borders. Frogs' legs, sheeps' eyes, larks' tongues and snails are delicacies which do not have universal appeal, nor, for that matter, do some of the regional dishes which are popular in some parts of our own country find favour in other areas. Tripe, haggis and cowheel are examples which come readily to mind. What we call 'acquired tastes' can, however, be changed without very much difficulty, as the tremendous expansion of foreign travel has demonstrated quite clearly in recent years.

The changes entailed by our search for optimum nutrition and freedom from the burden of ill health are fortunately not very formidable. In the main, what is required is a shift of emphasis — a balancing process calling merely for a reduction in the consumption of some types of food and a corresponding increase in others.

In the typical diet which we have already outlined in this chapter the main emphasis has been on starches and sugars (carbohydrates), meat and dairy produce (proteins), and fats, all of which leave acid by-products in the system when digested and assimilated, and so pave the way for the breakdown of body chemistry which leads first to acute illness and eventually to the insidious degenerative processes which characterize chronic disease.

Therefore, having allowed the body to carry out an effective 'spring-cleaning' process, it is necessary to ensure that the nutritional emphasis is shifted away from the acid-forming foods and to increase our consumption of the alkalizing elements provided by the vitamin- and mineral-rich fruits, vegetables and salads. Furthermore, we must ensure that the valuable nutrients which these foods provide are preserved to the greatest possible extent by either eating them raw or using conservative cooking procedures, about which we shall have more to say later (page 97).

The Vegetarian Diet

A rule-of-thumb balance which is widely accepted by naturopaths requires that the diet shall consist of 60 per cent of the alkaline fruits, vegetables and salads, and not more than 20 per cent each of the acid-forming carbohydrates and proteins. The latter will provide more than enough fats to meet the relatively low physiological requirements.

Such a regimen provides all the nutritional elements which the body requires for optimum sustenance, but we have still to bear in mind what has been said already concerning the *quality* of the foods which constitute our meals. In this context, it is relevant to discuss briefly the respective merits and demerits of a vegetarian diet as compared with one which includes meat and other animal derivatives.

The moral and humanitarian aspects of this very controversial subject have generated an enormous amount of public interest and concern in recent years, and there is no doubt that there has been very widespread revulsion against the battery system of food production. While we may personally applaud and support the various organisations which are concerned with conservation and humanitarian interests, our concern here is solely with health and nutritional considerations. Even orthodox nutritionists have long-since conceded that meat is not an essential constituent of the human diet and that lacto-vegetarian proteins are an adequate alternative dietary component.

Most naturopaths would go further and maintain that the human digestive system and our pattern of dentition is ill adapted for the consumption of meat, and that because of its acid nature and its liability to produce putrefactive residues in the intestines it should have little or no place in a health-promoting dietary.

Human teeth are designed primarily to grind the food we eat, whereas the purpose of those of carnivorous animals is to tear flesh from the bones of its prey and swallow it with virtually no premastication.

There is an equally wide variation in the digestive organs of the two groups, in that the chemical structure of the carnivore's gastric secretions is more specifically suited to the assimilation of flesh and bone, the residues of which are then more rapidly excreted through an intestinal tract which is substantially shorter than that of a man.

In addition to the physiological arguments against meat as a component of the human diet, there is no longer any doubt that when, as is too often the case, animal proteins constitute a major part of the food intake they can be responsible for a number of serious health hazards. There has been a great deal of press publicity in recent years in regard to the belief that there is a strong link between the amount of animal fat consumed and susceptibility to coronary heart disease. What is not so well known, however, is that a high-protein diet imposes a heavy strain on the kidneys, and this may well be a factor, therefore, in the increasing emphasis on the need for kidney transplants, even in relatively young people.

An excessive fat consumption also imposes considerable strain on the liver and gall-bladder, and since meat such as pork, mutton, and bacon can have a very high fat content — as much as 50 per cent in some cases — it is not difficult to see why moderation is so important in regard to the consumption of these food items.

It is not necessary, in the context of this book, to discuss at any length the complex and controversial distinction between saturated fats and unsaturated fats. Suffice it to say that the majority of the former are of animal origin, while most vegetable fats come within the unsaturated category. Current thinking is that it is the saturated animal fats which are most likely to contribute to health problems, whereas the unsaturated vegetable fats are more efficiently metabolized and therefore less harmful.

Having said that, however, it must be stressed that fat is a nutrient which is normally present only in relatively small proportions in natural wholefoods, and we should recognize in this fact a clear indication that fats should never be consumed except in extreme moderation as part of a balanced dietary. It explains, also, why fried and other fatty dishes should be avoided, and why butter, margarine, cream, salad oils, peanut butter and even some varieties of cheese should be taken only in the strictest moderation.

As a further cautionary warning regarding the extent to which the natural nutritional balance of popular foods can be distorted by the manufacturers, it will perhaps surprise many readers to learn that 'digestive' biscuits contain 20 per cent fat and 4 per cent salt; sweet mixed biscuits 31 per cent fat and 2 per cent salt; cream crackers 33 per cent fat and 4 per cent salt, while potato crisps — so beloved by children — contain $37\frac{1}{2}$ per cent fat and $3\frac{1}{2}$ per cent salt!

Bearing in mind what we have said concerning wholeness and balance as the basis for arranging a healthful diet, we can summarize our conclusions by reiterating that 60 per cent of our food should consist of fruit, vegetables and salads to meet the bulk of our vitamin, mineral and fibre needs as well as provide some easily assimilated fruit sugar and wholesome fluid; a further 20 per cent is comprised of wholegrain cereals in the form of wholewheat bread, muesli, rye or wholewheat crispbread, brown unpolished rice and wholewheat pastas.

The remaining 20 per cent will provide the protein element — perhaps some meat for those who do not wish to rely solely on vegetarian foods, but preferably dishes based on dairy products such as eggs and cheese, nuts, and pulses such as peas, beans, soya, etc.

It should be understood, however, that few of the items listed in the two latter groups are pure carbohydrates or proteins. Wholewheat flour, for example, is primarily a carbohydrate (73 per cent), but it also has a 9 per cent protein content and 2 per cent fat in the form of wheat-germ oil, while haricot beans, which are categorized as a protein, actually have a 45 per cent carbohydrate content.

As we have stressed repeatedly, it is not necessary to concern ourselves too meticulously with the *quantitative* element in dietetics provided that we observe the basic and far more important strictures concerning moderation, balance and *quality*.

These, then, are the mainstays of the naturopathic approach to the problems of tinnitus and catarrhal deafness — a clear understanding of the mechanics of hearing and the nature and causes of the congestion and inflammation which disorganize the functions of the ears, the initial cleansing process utilizing a short period of fasting in order to eliminate toxins from the blood and other bodily tissues, and then the use of sound nutrition to rebuild impaired tissues and restore normal organic functions.

These are the basic tools and modalities which are used in order to promote natural healing, but in order to reinforce them and ensure the speediest possible response and lasting efficacy there are other measures which need to be employed, and some commonly accepted practices which can have unsuspected harmful side-effects and which therefore have to be avoided or changed.

9.

Keep Moving

We referred briefly in Chapter 5 to the vital role which the lymphatic system plays in cleansing the bloodstream of toxic substances and we explained that the efficiency with which it is able to perform its important functions depends very largely on the alternate contraction and relaxation of the muscles which propels the lymph through the lymphatic ducts. Once this fact is appreciated it is easy to understand why the incidence of congestive and degenerative conditions such as catarrh, sinusitis, bronchitis and hardening of the arteries has increased so dramatically during the past half-century.

It is during this time that technical innovation and mechanical ingenuity have combined to produce machines and equipment which increasingly have served to remove the need for physical effort and thus encouraged a way of life in which muscular exercise can be largely dispensed with. The car and the television set are undoubtedly the major culprits in this respect.

Lack of Exercise
No more than a generation ago most people

depended on their legs to a large extent to reach places of employment, to visit friends, or go to sports grounds, cinemas and other places of entertainment. At weekends, millions of people of all ages set out on foot or on bicycles to reach local beauty spots and enjoy a few hours in the open air and, even for those who took advantage of public transport facilities, a walk — or run — to the railway station or bus or tram stop was a necessary preliminary.

Nowadays, car ownership is so widespread that for many people the daily round involves nothing more strenuous than a walk of a few yards to the car, another short walk from the car park to the office, shop or factory, a lunch-time stroll to the canteen, restaurant or pub, and then a reversal of the morning journey at the end of the day. After the evening meal, the usual routine will be to switch on the television and settle back into a comfortable chair until bedtime.

The objectives may change at the weekend, but the means of achieving them are often equally undemanding in terms of physical effort. In the summer, unless the lawn needs to be mowed or some other garden or household chore needs attention, it is likely that the family car will take the trail to the coast or out into the countryside. Once there, a bathe or stroll along the beach or through the woods may be undertaken, but many families will simply put out their deck-chairs or a blanket on the sands or grass and relax until the time comes to head for home.

Although the proliferation of labour-saving

domestic equipment has reduced the physical demands entailed in running a household, many housewives undoubtedly lead a more active life than their husbands and this may to some extent at least help to explain the phenomenon that women tend to live longer than men.

But the most serious cause for concern regarding the nation's health today undoubtedly lies in the fact that the pattern of inactivity is being laid down at an increasingly early age. Thanks to the family car and municipal transport, children are no longer required to walk to and from school in many cases, and even those who wish to take part in active recreations such as swimming, football, tennis, etc. are often driven to the venue by their parents who, understandably, are reluctant to expose them to the hazards of walking or cycling on crowded roads — and the even greater risks of molestation or worse.

For many youngsters today, addiction to the evening television programmes keeps them glued to the set until bedtime when they might otherwise be playing out of doors.

It would not be surprising, therefore, to find that the number of days lost from school because of colds, throat infections and other acute illnesses has increased considerably over the past decade or two, despite the higher living standards and the improvements in social conditions generally.

There is no doubt whatever that lack of physical exercise combined with the erosion of nutritional standards in regard to the nation's food is a major factor in the alarming increase in the incidence of deaths from heart disease and strokes. The considerable publicity given to this fact in recent years has, as is so often the case in human affairs, triggered a reaction among some sections of the population, but again as is not unusual, there has been a tendency to go from one extreme to another. Men and women of all ages, from schoolchildren to octogenarians, alerted to the need for exercise to maintain health and fitness, first seized upon jogging as a means of regaining or increasing their physical potential and then, beguiled by the nationwide publicity and a desire to raise funds for charity, allowed themselves to be caught up in the mass-marathon craze which has swept the world.

It is yet another tribute to the resilience of the human body and its capacity to withstand an extraordinary burden of physical abuse that thousands of those who set out on these exacting and awesome feats of endurance actually succeed in completing the course, but at what cost to their physical health in later life may never be known.

We have referred to these injudicious and potentially harmful extremes of physical activity merely to emphasize a very important principle which should be applied in *all* fields of human activity — physical, mental, nutritional, political and religious — namely, that extremes invariably invite suffering and retribution, and that *moderation* provides the only sure way to health, happiness and fulfilment.

Therefore, in considering the types of exercise which need to be undertaken to promote health and well-being our aim will be to ensure that the muscles shall be kept supple and responsive to normal demands, the circulation of both blood and lymph shall be stimulated regularly and adequately, and that the joints shall be encouraged to move freely through as wide a range as possible. For older people in particular, and for those who for any reason are in a poor physical condition, caution is essential at the outset in order to avoid imposing undue strain on either muscles, joints or vital organs.

Walking

The exercise which meets most of our needs and which avoids most of the pitfalls is undoubtedly the one which our bodies are designed to undertake — namely, walking. The upright posture which man has adopted in the process of evolution has given rise to a number of anatomical and physiological problems, one of the most serious of which is that of maintaining an efficient circulation of blood and lymph throughout the body. The healthy heart is a very efficient pump which has no difficulty in propelling freshly oxygenated blood through the arteries to all the extremities and upward to the brain, but there is no such propulsive power to effect the return flow via the veins and lymph vessels. To achieve this task of maintaining a constant circulation from the extremities and abdominal organs against the pull of gravity the body has to rely on the rhythmic contraction and relaxation of the muscles surrounding the veins, and it is for this reason that walking is such a valuable exercise.

It mobilizes not only all the muscles of the

feet, legs, thighs and abdomen as well as those of the arms and shoulders, but also induces regular deep-breathing. The resultant expansion and relaxation of the ribs and lungs, combined with the rise and fall of the muscular diaphragm, sucks the blood first into the abdomen from the large veins of the thighs, then into the chest cavity and so back to the heart, while at the same time the lymph is propelled upwards to be returned to the main circulatory system via the veins at the base of the neck.

Walking achieves all this with the utmost economy of effort and without the need for expensive or complicated equipment. Not only can it be fitted conveniently into the daily routine of people of all ages but it can actually effect a not inconsiderable saving in monetary terms in many cases, and also broaden one's social horizons. It has been said with considerable justification that anyone who feels cut off and isolated from human contacts need only acquire either a baby or a dog — preferably both — and go for a short walk. It is unlikely that he or she will have ventured far without being halted by someone who wishes to admire the baby or pat the dog!

Those who use a car or public transport to reach their place of employment can avail themselves of the benefits of pedestrianism simply by leaving the car, bus or train a suitable distance from their destination and completing the journey on foot. Housewives, too, can insist on walking their children to school or leaving the car at home when they go shopping or visiting friends. Here, again, what is needed is simply the establishment of a new set of habit patterns to allow for the necessary adjustment in the daily timetable.

It is not only the circulatory system that benefits from physical activity. The muscles become stronger and more resilient, the mobility of the joints is progressively increased, and the deeper breathing which is induced helps to reduce any catarrhal congestion in the nose, sinuses and lungs. A further bonus can be achieved if, when walking, one makes a conscious effort to straighten the spine, which in turn will mean pulling in the abdomen and so gradually reducing any distension around the waistline.

Neck Mobility

Sufferers from tinnitus and catarrhal deafness, in particular, should make a point, when walking, of turning the head as far as possible to look over the shoulder from time to time, when crossing the road for example. This simple exercise will gradually break down adhesions in the neck and upper spine and improve mobility in that important area, impairment of which is often a contributory factor in these ear disorders. It is all too easy, over the years, to get into the habit of turning the whole body on these occasions with the result that the head is seldom rotated to anything approaching the full extent of which it should be capable. Consequently, the muscles and ligaments tend to become increasingly shortened and thickened, which in turn leads to restriction of the blood-supply to the head and the sensory organs located therein, including, of course, the eyes, the brain and the ears.

Nor is this the only impediment resulting from reduced mobility in the neck and upper spine, for the main nerve-trunks from the brain are concentrated in this area, through which are transmitted the nerve impulses which control such vital organs as the heart, the lungs and the digestive system. Tension and constriction in this part of the body, therefore, may well have far-reaching detrimental effects on the health of the body as a whole.

Because the loss of mobility in the neck is such an insidious and gradual process few people are aware of the deterioration until they are required to carry out a few simple tests. For example, most middle-aged and older people will have difficulty in turning the head sufficiently to enable them to identify someone standing three or four metres directly behind them while keeping the shoulders immobile. Similarly, tension and stiffness in the neck will be revealed by the emission of creaking and crackling noises when the head is rotated in such a way that the nose performs a wide circling movement.

Sufferers from tinnitus and catarrhal deafness should therefore be aware of the need to restore the maximum possible degree of mobility in this vital area of the spine, not only for the purpose of gaining the maximum possible improvement in regard to their immediate problems but also because the upper spine is one of the areas where stress and tension can be the precursor of subsequent arthritic changes. Therefore, both for the immediate benefits which may be achieved and as an insurance against future rheumatic degenerative changes it is imperative that remedial action be taken without delay in all cases where impaired neck mobility is detected.

There is no doubt that the speediest possible progress will be made in this respect if the services of an experienced osteopath can be enlisted. Not only will he be able to assess the extent and nature of any specific spinal lesions, but in addition to carrying out corrective adjustments he will also manipulate the muscles and other soft tissues with the object of breaking down adhesions, and counsel his patient regarding appropriate remedial exercises and relaxation techniques which are likely to be helpful. Those who, for any reason, are unable to avail themselves of professional help can, however, do a great deal to improve neck mobility by practising regularly and conscientiously a series of simple exercises such as those described in Appendix B on pages 119–23.

It is important, also, to avoid allowing the shoulders to sag and the head to drop forward — a postural defect which characterizes so many people from middle age onwards. Here, again, the establishment of the correct habit-pattern is required, the aim being to carry the head high at all times, keeping the shoulders squared but relaxed, the knees braced and the abdomen firm and taut so that the curve of the lower spine is not allowed to become exaggerated. At night, the head should be supported comfortably on one or two soft pillows only sufficiently high as to avoid excessive sideways or forward flexion of the neck when lying either on one side or the back.

The importance of spinal flexibility and mobility cannot be overemphasized because, as was frequently stressed by the late Albert Rumfitt — one of our most experienced and talented osteopaths — 'the spine is the first organ of the human body to undergo the degenerative changes of the aging process'. Therefore, whatever we can do to minimize the effects of wear and tear on this vital structure will pay incalculable dividends in terms of our future health and physical well-being.

Central Heating

If defective nutrition and reduced physical activity are the two primary causes of the circulatory and lymphatic congestion which predispose to catarrhal conditions such as tinnitus and deafness, the third most harmful factor must surely be the revolutionary changes which have taken place in regard to domestic heating systems over the past two or three decades. Today, some form of central heating is regarded as an essential feature of every new house or flat that is built, and even in relatively old properties the traditional open fire has been replaced by a gas or oil-fired boiler or electric storage heaters. In terms of personal comfort this change has undoubtedly proved to be of incalculable benefit, but little or no thought has been given to its effects on the human circulatory system.

The installation of a thermostatically-controlled heating system in the house has to a considerable extent rendered redundant and inoperative the body's own ingenious heat-control mechanisms. It is undoubtedly true that, so far as human anatomy and physiology are concerned, 'what we do not use we lose,' and when we cocoon ourselves in an atmosphere of unvarying warmth and comfort our circulatory system quickly loses the capacity to adjust speedily and efficiently to changes in external temperature.

The practice of clothing ourselves in order to conserve heat has long since caused us to lose the protective covering of bodily hair, but the circulatory system can still function as a very efficient thermostat which can cool the bloodstream in hot weather and retain internal heat during the cold winter months. Thus, as soon as the internal temperature of the body rises appreciably above the norm of 37°C (98.4°F) the capillaries just beneath the skin expand so that a larger volume of blood is drawn to the surface and exposed to the cooling influence of the atmosphere, aided by increased perspiration which dissipates heat by vaporization. Simultaneously, the blood supply to the lungs is increased to be cooled by the inhalation of colder air. Conversely, when the temperature falls, the surface tissues of the body contract (the 'goose-pimple' effect) forcing blood from the superficial capillaries into the deeper tissues so that heat loss is minimized. Under conditions of extreme cold the body resorts to another ingenious means of generating internal heat by inducing involuntary muscular activity in the form of shivering. These complex mechanisms will, however, cease to function efficiently if they are not kept in constant use, which means exposing the body to frequent variations in temperature.

The modern trend towards warmer clothing, efficient home-heating and insulation, and the use of heated car transport has effectively shielded many of us from all but relatively minor changes of temperature, with the result that the skin and superficial blood-vessels remain in a state of constant warmth and relaxation throughout the day and night.

Moreover, the food which serves as fuel to generate bodily heat consists very largely of the high-calorie starches and sugars, and because we go to such lengths to conserve heat by external means the body is not required to burn up much of this fuel, the residues of which are increasingly deposited in the deeper tissues. As a consequence, individuals who have a 'slow-burning' low metabolic rate tend to become overweight, while those with a more active metabolism are likely to accumulate the surplus material in the form of catarrhal mucus.

The reader will, therefore, understand why, in order to clear the tissues of these unwanted residues as quickly and efficiently as possible, we advise not only regular, vigorous exercise combined with deep breathing, but also the avoidance of excessive indulgence in hot baths, the use of hot water for washing purposes, and even the inclusion of very hot foods and drinks in the diet.

Because hot water is so readily available nowadays it is a very common practice to take a hot bath or shower daily — a practice which induces circulatory congestion and weakens the skin and superficial blood-vessels. To reverse this effect, therefore, and strengthen the skin and blood-vessels while at the same time stimulating the circulation and relieving localised congestion, it is necessary merely to wash only in cool or cold water — preferably using a mild herbal or vegetable soap — and to have a cool or cold sponge-down or shower each morning followed by a brisk friction-rub using a skin-brush or very coarse towel. A moderately hot bath may be taken once weekly, but this also should be followed by the sponge-down and friction-rub.

This may seem a somewhat heroic practice initially, but once the new habit-pattern has become established it will be found that the stimulus provided by the cold water and the friction induces a delicious warm glow throughout the body which is in pleasant contrast to the chill often experienced after hot water has been used.

10.

On Your Marks, Get Set...

In the next chapter we shall set out a detailed, stage-by-stage treatment programme, but before doing so we must explain briefly certain recurring procedures which will be employed from time to time.

The Short Fast
During the initial cleansing fast it is imperative that no solid food of any kind is taken, since the object of this procedure is to rest the digestive and assimilative systems and allow the body to concentrate all its energies on the elimination from the deeper tissues of unwanted or harmful residues. The embargo applies also to milk foods and beverages, fruit and vegetable purées, soups and broths, bottled 'fruit squashes', tea and coffee.

Only fresh tap-water, or one of the bottled mineral waters, or freshly pressed fruit or vegetable juices may be taken, the latter diluted with an equal quantity of fresh water and sipped slowly. Pure, unsweetened apple, grape and other fruit and vegetable juices are obtainable from health food stores, but if a hand-press or electric juicer is available it is better to extract fresh juice and drink it immediately. Do not be tempted to drink excessively with the mistaken idea of 'flushing out the system' — a procedure which will merely impose an unnecessary work-load on the kidneys and so dissipate vital energy needed for eliminative purposes. Only sufficient fluid should be taken to satisfy natural thirst — preferably small quantities at a time.

Rest as much as possible, both physically and mentally, during the day, and try to retire early to allow a minimum of eight hours' sleep.

The Cleansing Diet

Following the short fast, the tissue-cleansing process must be sustained, for which purpose a restricted diet consisting only of fresh fruit should be taken for the next three days, interspersed with drinks of water or dilute juices as needed.

Continue to rest as much as possible, but a walk out of doors, combined with deep breathing, or some other gentle exercise, may be taken with advantage provided that it does not tax physical resources unduly. Older people for whom rheumatism is a problem should maintain as high a degree of physical mobility as possible. It is also advisable in these cases to omit oranges from the diet, as well as lemons and grapefruit and their juices, but otherwise it is a good plan to vary the fruit meals as much as possible, not only to avoid monotony but to ensure that the widest possible range of vitamins, trace elements and other nutrients is maintained.

With the reservation concerning rheumatic sufferers, each fruit meal may consist of one or more of the following varieties: apples, pears, grapes, melon, oranges, grapefruit, peaches, pineapples, or any other juicy fruit in season, but no bananas, tinned or bottled fruit or dried or stewed fruit.

The Maintenance Diet

Once the cleansing régime has been completed, the next consideration is to provide a balanced diet of simple whole foods which will reactivate the digestive and assimilative organs and provide all the essential nutrients needed by the body to restore chemical equilibrium, maintain organic functions and provide the vital energy required to sustain muscular activities.

On the basis of the 60:20:20 ratio outlined in Chapter 8, the mainstay of the diet will be the alkaline fruits and vegetables, but some discretion needs to be exercised by those (particularly older people) whose previous diet has largely excluded raw vegetables, salads and wholegrain cereals. The sudden introduction of relatively large amounts of these foods, with their high-fibre content, can present the digestive system with problems with which it is not equipped to cope. The result may well be indigestion, flatulence, abdominal distension and constipation. The risk of any such eventuality will be minimized if our earlier injunction is observed — namely, to take only relatively small meals, eat slowly and masticate thoroughly.

If, however, digestive problems arise despite

these precautions, the wholegrain cereals, salads, and raw vegetable elements in the diet should be reduced temporarily, and replaced with conservatively cooked vegetables, soaked or stewed dried or fresh fruits, and bread made from a lower extraction flour. This means choosing a loaf described as 'wheatmeal', 'farmhouse', 'granary', etc., which are euphemisms for brown bread which is not made from 100 per cent wholemeal flour. (Incidentally, when purchasing 100 per cent wholemeal bread it is necessary to insist on the description 'wholemeal' or 'wholewheat', because by law these terms may not be applied to bread made from lower extraction flour. Moreover, bread so described is free from the synthetic vitamins and minerals — e.g. chalk and iron — which by law must be added to *all* bread made from lower-extraction flour.)

The amount of raw food and wholegrain cereals should be increased gradually as the digestive system becomes accustomed to the wholefood diet.

The need for conservative cooking is stressed in order to guard against the nutritional losses incurred when vegetables and other foods are boiled in the conventional manner. Casseroling and steaming ensure that such losses are kept to a minimum, although the use of a pressure cooker is permissible provided that the maker's cooking times are observed meticulously. Because of the very high temperatures involved in this method, the slightest degree of over-cooking can greatly increase the destruction of certain nutrients.

Specimen menus are given in Appendix A on pages 113–18, but readers who are not familiar with the principles of healthful feeding would be well advised to obtain one of the excellent wholefood cookery manuals issued by the publishers of this book, from whom a catalogue of suitable titles may be obtained on request. A selection of these publications will be found on the shelves of most health food stores and good bookshops.

Baths

We have already stressed the harmful effects of over-indulgence in hot baths, and explained why cool or cold water is beneficial both in stimulating the blood and lymph circulation and toning up the skin. For this reason the daily sponge-down and friction-rub is an important component in the treatment plan.

It is a simple procedure requiring only the use of a large, thick face-flannel — approximately 10 inches (25cm) square — and a large rough towel. A bath-brush with a long handle is a useful alternative to the flannel.

The flannel or brush is dipped in cold water, the surplus being wrung or shaken out, and then the face, shoulders, arms, trunk and legs are vigorously sponged or brushed, not forgetting the spine. The whole process need occupy no more than a minute or two, after which the body is rubbed vigorously with the towel until it is dry. The exercise and the friction both combine to generate heat and leave the body glowing.

Compresses

Cold water can also be used to relieve localized

congestion and inflammation and at the same time stimulate the circulation to the affected tissues, thus hastening the process of recovery.

For this purpose, a combined neck and chest compress is used. The neck compress consists of strips of cotton or linen material (old sheets can be used) about 15 inches (38cm) in length and 4 inches (10cm) in width when folded two or three times. This material is wrung out well in cold water, wrapped around the neck and then covered with a slightly wider layer of dry woollen material the end of which is secured by a safety-pin or adhesive tape.

The chest compress is made up and applied in the same way, but the material will, of course, need to be wider and longer (10 inches/25cm wide when folded, and 36 inches/90cm in length). When the chest compress is used it is a good plan to place a hot-water bottle at the feet.

The compresses should remain in position for at least two hours, but for maximum effect they should be applied just before retiring and kept in place all night. A pleasant, warm reaction should be experienced within a few minutes of application, and the compresses should have dried out completely by the time they are removed, when the skin should be sponged down and dried thoroughly. The compress material should be washed before being reapplied.

If the body does not warm up, the compress should be removed and reapplied the next day.

Clearing Wax Obstruction

If there is reason to suspect that wax has

accumulated in the outer ear, steps should be taken to clear it as soon as possible. Syringing is the most effective method of removal, but it should be carried out only by an experienced practitioner.

Failing this, it is often possible to soften the wax and remove it gradually by mixing six drops of almond oil with six drops of hydrogen peroxide solution. A small spoon should be warmed in hot water and dried. The oil mixture is then put into it and allowed to warm slightly. With the head resting on a cushion or pillow, a few drops are then trickled into the ear which is pulled and massaged gently to ensure maximum penetration. After retaining the oil for about ten to fifteen minutes a twist of soft cotton or linen material is inserted gently into the ear to soak up the surplus and remove some of the softened wax.

If the treatment is carried out just before retiring a small plug of cotton material should be inserted and left in position until the following morning, an old towel being folded and laid on the pillow to prevent the latter from being soiled.

On no account should cotton-wool be inserted, nor should the ear be probed with a match-stick or any similar hard instrument.

From time to time during the day it is a good plan to grasp the ear-lobe between the first and middle fingers and massage around the base of the ear, pressing gently and moving the finger-tips in a circle.

Inflating the Eustachian Tube

A useful means of easing congestion in the

Eustachian tube is to pinch the nostrils between the fingers, close the mouth and attempt to blow the nose. Unless the tube is completely blocked this should result in a 'swishing' noise in the ear and the ear-drum will be felt to move in response to the increase in air-pressure.

A similar but less pronounced effect can be produced by yawning vigorously four or five times — a simple exercise which can be practised repeatedly with benefit throughout the day.

Avoid Irritants

Inflammation of the throat, Eustachian tube and middle ear can be aggravated and to some extent perpetuated by the inhalation of irritant dust and fumes and exposure to draughts of cold air. Every effort should be made, therefore, to avoid localized chilling such as may occur when sitting in a draughty room or near an open window when travelling in a car, bus or train.

The harm which can be caused by the heat and fumes as a result of inhaling tobacco smoke is now so widely recognized that it should not be necessary here to urge cigarette and pipe smokers to take steps to break the habit without delay.

Other chemical irritants which should be avoided as far as possible are petrol and exhaust fumes, aerosol sprays, hair lacquer, nail varnish and removers, and fumes given off by household paints and emulsions.

It is appreciated that all these injunctions may appear initially to be complex and even confusing, but as is the case with many new concepts, familiarity quickly establishes comprehension and the reader is urged, therefore, to reread the preceding pages before embarking on the detailed treatment plan which we are now ready to set forth.

11.

...Go!

The following treatment schedule includes aii the therapeutic measures which have been explained at length in the preceding pages, together with the neck-mobilization exercises which are described and illustrated in Appendix B on pages 119–23.

Clearly, however, business and domestic commitments will dictate the extent to which individual readers will be able to keep to the suggested daily timetables, and it is permissible, therefore, to vary the sequence of events as circumstances require, provided always that the dietetic restrictions are strictly observed. For example, it may be more convenient to have a cooked meal at midday, in which case the salad, fruit or other raw dishes may be taken in the evening. Similarly, if there are pressing commitments in the morning, the wax-removal procedure and/or neck exercises may have to be omitted provided, of course, that they are carried out conscientiously later in the day, or before retiring.

Outdoor exercise, also, should be fitted into the day's routine as conveniently as possible.

It is emphasized, however, that the following

schedule is planned for optimum effectiveness, and every effort should be made, therefore, to keep to the suggested programme. In long-standing and severe cases it may be necessary to repeat the full schedule in two months' time, and so it is suggested that a record of the date of commencement be kept for reference purposes.

Day 1

1. *On rising:* Glass of water or dilute fresh fruit or vegetable juice sipped slowly. No solid foods or other liquids of any kind throughout the day.

   Moderately hot bath and/or tepid or cold sponge-down followed by friction-rub.

2. Oil and hydrogen peroxide treatment for wax removal if needed (see page 100).

3. Neck mobilization exercises (see pages 119–23).

4. Outdoor exercise if possible — for example a brisk half-hour walk combined with deep breathing. On return, sponge-down and friction-rub; change of clothing if necessary.

5. Drink of water or dilute juice if needed.

6. Rest for half hour if possible.

7. Normal activities as necessary, but avoid as far as possible anything involving undue physical or mental strain. Rest from time to time and take drinks as needed.

8. *Early evening:* Outdoor exercise if possible. Drink if needed.

9. *Before retiring:* Wax-removal treatment if

necessary. Drink if needed.

Apply neck and chest compresses (see page 99) and retire to bed early in a darkened but ventilated room. If for any reason it is not desirable to leave a window ajar, the bedroom door should remain at least partially open.

Days 2 and 3

Repeat Day 1 schedule, but if feeling lethargic or experiencing headache or other 'healing' crisis' symptoms forgo or reduce the outdoor exercise sessions and try to have more rest, preferably in a darkened room.

Day 4

1. *On rising:* Glass of water or dilute juice sipped slowly.
   Tepid or cold sponge-down and friction-rub.

2. Wax-removal treatment if necessry.

3. Neck-mobilization exercises.

4. *Breakfast:* Fresh fruit only (approximately 1 lb/455g), for example an apple, a pear and a few grapes. Do not be tempted to overeat.

5. Outdoor exercise if desired, followed by sponge-down and friction-rub.

6. Take drinks of water or dilute juice between meals as needed.

7. *Midday:* Fruit as for breakfast, but quantity may be increased to approximately $1\frac{1}{2}$ lb (680g).

8. Normal activities as necessary, interspersed with rest periods when possible.

9. *Early evening:* Fruit as at midday.
   Outdoor exercise, if desired, followed by sponge-down and friction-rub — preferably before the meal or not less than one hour afterwards.

10. *Before retiring:* Wax-removal treatment if necessary. Neck mobilization exercises, sponge-down and friction-rub.

Days 5 and 6
Repeat Day 4 schedule, but apply compresses only on 5th night.

Unless very lethargic, try to have *some* outdoor exercise.

Day 7
Adapt the following programme as necessary to fit in with normal commitments.

1. *On rising:* Glass of water or dilute juice sipped slowly.
   Sponge-down and friction-rub.

2. Wax-removal treatment if necessary.

3. Neck-mobilization exercises.

4. *Breakfast:* Any fresh fruit as on preceding days, *or* stewed apple or other fruit, *or* dried fruit either stewed or soaked overnight. Also $\frac{1}{4}$ pint (140ml) natural unflavoured yogurt.

5. Outdoor exercise if possible, followed by sponge-down and friction-rub.

6. Drinks of water or dilute juice between meals as needed.

7. *Midday:* As for breakfast.

8. Outdoor exercise followed by sponge-down and friction-rub, preferably before the evening meal or not less than one hour afterwards.

9. *Evening meal:* Small mixed salad of lettuce, tomato, watercress, grated raw carrot and 1 oz (30g) of washed raisins or sultanas. An apple, pear or a few grapes if desired.

10. *Before retiring:* Wax removal if necessary. Neck mobilization exercises, sponge-down and friction-rub.

Day 8

Repeat Day 7 schedule but have weekly hot bath followed by sponge-down and friction-rub.

Days 9 and 10

1. *On rising:* Glass of water or dilute juice sipped slowly.
   Sponge-down and friction-rub.

2. Discontinue wax-removal treatment as soon as outer ear is clear.

3. Neck-mobilization exercises.

4. *Breakfast:* Fruit as on preceding days with yogurt.

5. Outdoor exercise if possible followed by sponge-down and friction-rub.

6. Drinks of water or dilute juice between meals as needed.

7. *Midday:* As for breakfast.

8. Outdoor exercise followed by sponge-down and friction-rub before evening meal or one hour afterwards.

9. *Evening meal:* Small mixed salad as on preceding days, but with the addition of 1 oz (30g) grated nuts and one slice of wholewheat bread or crispbread spread very thinly with vegetable margarine, followed by an apple, pear or other fruit if desired.

10. *Before retiring:* Neck mobilization exercises.
    Sponge-down and friction-rub.

Days 11 to 14
As preceding days except:

Midday: Salad as previous evening meal.

Evening meal: A serving of conservatively cooked vegetables — for example cabbage, carrots and onions (no potatoes) — with a lightly poached egg, *or* a little lean meat, *or* 1 oz (30g) grated cheese. Fresh fruit, *or* baked apple, *or* soaked or simmered dried fruit.

Day 15 Onwards

1. *On rising:* Glass of water or dilute juice.
   Sponge-down and friction rub.

2. *Breakfast:* See menus in Appendix A (pages 113–18).

3. Drinks as needed between meals. A cup or two of weak unsweetened tea or decaffeinated

coffee may be taken in place of usual drinks.

4. *Midday:* See menus.

5. Outdoor exercise should be taken at any convenient time during the day, extending to a total of one hour's duration when possible, and followed by sponge-down and friction-rub.

6. *Evening Meal:* See menus.

7. *Before retiring:* Neck exercises and sponge-down and friction-rub.

Afterword

On completion of the initial course of treatment it is necessary to maintain a simple, health-promoting life-style based on the Day 15 schedule in order to consolidate the cleansing and restorative processes which have been set in motion. Progress towards full recovery will inevitably vary from one individual to another depending upon such factors as age, health history, physical resources, and the duration and severity of the symptoms. A progressive improvement should, however, be experienced in most cases in the course of three months from the commencement of the treatment programme. In more obstinate cases, where full recovery has not been achieved in that time, the full therapeutic régime should be repeated.

Patience and perseverence are the keystones to success in our efforts to eliminate physical and functional defects which in many cases will have developed insidiously as a result of many years of bodily misuse and faulty nutrition. Remember that the reward for sustained effort is not merely relief from tinnitus and catarrhal deafness — desirable as this goal may be — but the achievement of the high standard of overall health, fitness and vitality which alone can ensure maximum immunity from acute and chronic disease.

Appendix A

A Week's Menus

The following menus are intended to illustrate the type of simple balanced meals which will meet 'normal' nutritional needs and satisfy most 'normal' appetites. Because, however, individual needs vary so widely according to such factors as age, sex, physical characteristics, occupational demands, sporting activities, etc. a reasonable degree of flexibility must be allowed in regard to the choice of foods, the amount consumed and the timing of meals, provided always that the overall balance is maintained in accordance with the 60:20:20 ratios explained on page 78, and that habitual overeating is avoided.

Moderation, not fanaticism, should be the guiding principle in regard to all aspects of healthful living.

In particular, white flour and sugar, and the many processed foods containing these denatured commodities, should be assiduously avoided, as also should milk foods and beverages, salt and other condiments and strong tea, coffee and alcohol. Animal proteins — meat, fish and poultry — may be substituted by vegetarian dishes if desired, but fried and fatty foods should be avoided.

First Day

Breakfast: Muesli (see recipe on page 117).

Midday: Salad of lettuce, tomato, grated raw beetroot and watercress, with one slice of wholemeal toast (cold) spread thinly with peanut butter.

Evening: A mixed vegetable casserole sprinkled with 2 oz (55g) grated cheese. An apple, *or* a pear, *or* some grapes.

Second Day

Breakfast: Soaked or stewed dried fruit sprinkled with a dessertspoon of wheatgerm.

Midday: Lettuce and chopped celery dressed with cottage cheese. An orange, *or* a pear.

Evening: Two nut cutlets (mixture obtainable from health food stores) with steamed carrots and spinach. Baked apple stuffed with raisins.

Third Day

Breakfast: Half a grapefruit (sweetened if necessary with a little melted honey) and ¼ pint (140ml) natural yogurt.

Midday: Lightly poached egg on wholewheat toast. An apple or some grapes.

Evening: Ambrosia Salad (see recipe on page 117), with two slices of wholemeal bread or crispbread spread thinly with vegetarian margarine.

Fourth Day

Breakfast: Muesli (see page 117).

Midday: Lettuce, grated carrot, tomato, cucumber and 1 oz (30g) washed raisins or sultanas.

Evening: Plain omelette with steamed peas and potatoes (washed thoroughly and cooked in skins).
Fresh fruit salad.

Fifth Day

Breakfast: Stewed prunes sprinkled with a dessertspoon of wheatgerm.

Midday: Two slices of wholewheat toast or crispbread with cottage cheese. An apple *or* a pear.

Evening: Cauliflower cheese with jacket potato.
Sliced ripe banana in yogurt.

Sixth Day

Breakfast: Stewed apple with chopped dates and yogurt.

Midday: Scrambled egg on wholewheat toast.

Evening: Ambrosia Salad (see page 117).

Seventh Day

Breakfast: Fresh fruit salad and wheatgerm.

Midday: Lettuce, celery, sliced banana and yogurt.

Evening: Lean meat or poultry, or vegetarian savoury, with steamed potatoes (cooked in skins), cabbage and carrots.
Fruit crumble (made with wholemeal flour).

Notes

1. Any fruits, vegetables or salads which are not in season may be replaced by similar items. During the winter months, for example, chopped or grated carrots, beetroot, cabbage, sprouts, etc. may be used instead of summer vegetables.

2. Non-vegetarians may replace egg, cheese and nut dishes with 2 to 3 oz (55 to 85g) of lean meat, poultry or fish.

3. Fruit should always be fully ripe. Sour or unripe food should not be eaten either raw or cooked.

4. If cooked fruit needs to be sweetened a little honey may be added. White sugar should never be used.

5. Proprietary 'salad creams', salad dressings, sauces, table-salt and other condiments should never be added to food either during cooking or when served. If a salad dressing is desired it should consist of natural yogurt or no more than a dessertspoon of olive oil or

corn oil mixed with a teaspoon of lemon juice or orange juice. A little celery salt may be added to vegetables if desired.

Two Useful Recipes

MUESLI

Muesli can be used as a very nutritious breakfast dish or a light midday or evening meal.

1 heaped dessertspoon washed raisins, sultanas or chopped dates
2 or 3 heaped dessertspoons coarse oatmeal
1 level dessertspoon honey (optional)
4 dessertspoons warm water
½ medium apple
2 heaped dessertspoons grated nuts (peanuts, hazels or cashews, etc.)
½ ripe banana

1. Mix the dried fruit into the oatmeal.
2. Melt honey (if desired) in the warm water, pour over oatmeal and leave to soak for one hour or overnight.
3. Before serving add grated apple, sprinkle over grated nuts and decorate with banana slices.

AMBROSIA SALAD

This salad constitutes a very nutritious and satisfying meal and it can be prepared — and cleared — more quickly than most cooked meals.

If desired, it may be taken with one or two slices of wholemeal toast or crispbread spread thinly with yeast extract, peanut butter or honey.

Non-vegetarians may omit the apple and banana and substitute 2 oz (55g) lean meat, poultry or fish before adding the grated cheese and nuts.

Lettuce leaves
Tomato, sliced
Cucumber, sliced
Beetroot (raw or cooked — no vinegar) grated or
    sliced
½ medium apple
1 dessertspoon washed dried fruit (sultanas, raisins, chopped dates, etc.)
2 oz (55g) cheese
2 dessertspoons grated nuts (peanuts, hazels, cashews, etc.)
½ ripe banana

1. Tear the lettuce leaves into pieces and line a large plate, then decorate with sliced tomato and cucumber and grated or sliced beetroot.
2. Dice the apple into small pieces and scatter over, followed by the dried fruit.
3. Finally, grate the cheese and scatter over, followed by the grated nuts, and decorate with banana slices.

Appendix B

Neck Mobilization Exercises

The exercises illustrated here should be performed slowly and gently at first, without undue strain or any attempt to force the head and neck beyond the range which can be achieved comfortably, the aim being to increase gradually both the number of repetitions and the range of movement.

The intriguing creaks, crackles, clicks and other noises which may emerge from the joints as a result of the unaccustomed movements need cause no anxiety, and they should gradually diminish and eventually disappear as mobility is progressively improved.

Ideally, the exercises should be practised regularly night and morning, but otherwise any of them, or the whole sequence, can be fitted into the daily routine at any convenient opportunity. The complete series can be performed comfortably in little more than five minutes.

Note: The exercises should not be continued if pain is experienced when the head is rotated, and anyone suffering from an arthritic condition of the upper spine should seek professional advice before attempting them.

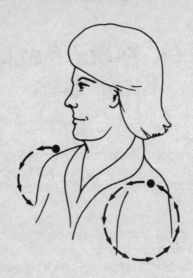

Exercise 1

1. Sit comfortably with hands resting lightly on thighs. Keeping the head still, raise both shoulders as high as possible, then hunch them forwards, drop them down and back, then up again to the starting position, so that the points of the shoulders have completed a smooth circling movement.

Relax for a few moments, then repeat from six to twelve times before reversing the direction of the shoulder movements for the same number of repetitions, relaxing momentarily between each.

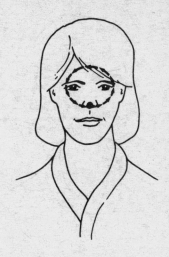

Exercise 2

2. Keeping the shoulders firmly against the back of the chair, move the head first to the right, then up, across to the left, down, and back to the starting position so that the nose describes a wide circle.

Repeat from six to twelve times, then relax for a few moments and repeat in the opposite direction.

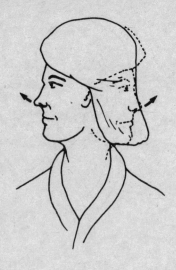

Exercise 3

3. Keeping the shoulders still, turn the head slowly to the right as far as it will go without strain, then to the left, repeating from six to twelve times.

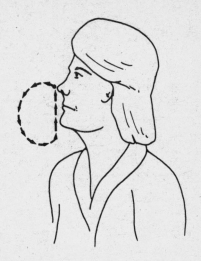

Exercise 4

4. Keeping the shoulders steady, raise the head and look up at the ceiling, then thrust it gently forward and downward until the chin rests on the front of the neck; finally, keeping the chin pulled back, raise the head to the starting position.

Repeat from six to twelve times, relax, and then repeat the same sequence of movements in the reverse direction.

INDEX

In the same series ...

HIGH BLOOD-PRESSURE

Explains a remarkably successful approach to this dangerous condition, which so often results in paralytic stroke or cerebral haemorrhage, incapacitating thousands of vital men and women in the prime of life. *Contents include:* Symptoms of High Blood-pressure; Wrong Diet is Enemy No. 1; Cholesterol Theory Proved Correct; Defective Kidneys and High Blood-pressure; Effects of Tobacco; Seven Corrective Principles; Meat-eating Fallacy; Foods on the Taboo List; Foods to be Cut Down; Vitamins and High Blood-pressure; Impressive Results with Vitamin E; The Rice Diet 'Cure'; Starved Nerves; A Toxic Blood Stream; Hardening of the Arteries; The Circulatory System.

VARICOSE VEINS

Varicose veins, varicose ulcers, haemorrhoids and phlebitis are all complaints directly arising from breakdown of the circulatory tissues. Injections and surgical removal can offer nothing more than temporary alleviation. In this book an experienced Nature Cure practitioner explains the causes of breakdown and provides self-treament methods by which the resultant disorders may be permanently overcome. *Contents include:* Cause of varicose ulcer; How varicosity arises — pregnancy, childbirth, obesity, weight loss, injury, fallen arches; Feeding the veins — specimen diets; The water cure; Constipation — enemas; Haemorrhoids (piles) — internal and external; Treatment for phlebitis.